Study Guide for

Wong's Essentials of Pediatric Nursing

Tenth Edition

Marilyn J. Hockenberry, PhD, RN, PPCNP-BC, FAAN
Bessie Baker Professor of Nursing and Professor of Pediatrics
Chair, Duke Institutional Review Board
Duke University
Durham, North Carolina

David Wilson, MS, RNC-NIC (deceased)
Staff
Children's Hospital at Saint Francis
Tulsa, Oklahoma

Cheryl C. Rodgers, PhD, RN, CPNP, CPON
Assistant Professor
Duke University School of Nursing
Durham, North Carolina

Prepared by

Cheryl C. Rodgers, PhD, RN, CPNP, CPON
Assistant Professor
Duke University School of Nursing
Durham, North Carolina

Kelley Ward, PhD, RNC
Freelance author/writer in the field of nursing and health care
Owasso, Oklahoma

ELSEVIER

ELSEVIER

3251 Riverport Lane
St. Louis, Missouri 63043

STUDY GUIDE FOR WONG'S ESSENTIALS OF
PEDIATRIC NURSING TENTH EDITION

ISBN: 978-0-323-42984-9

Notices

Knowledge and best practice in this field are constantly changing. As new research and experience broaden our understanding, changes in research methods, professional practices, or medical treatment may become necessary.

Practitioners and researchers must always rely on their own experience and knowledge in evaluating and using any information, methods, compounds, or experiments described herein. In using such information or methods they should be mindful of their own safety and the safety of others, including parties for whom they have a professional responsibility.

With respect to any drug or pharmaceutical products identified, readers are advised to check the most current information provided (i) on procedures featured or (ii) by the manufacturer of each product to be administered, to verify the recommended dose or formula, the method and duration of administration, and contraindications. It is the responsibility of practitioners, relying on their own experience and knowledge of their patients, to make diagnoses, to determine dosages and the best treatment for each individual patient, and to take all appropriate safety precautions.

To the fullest extent of the law, neither the Publisher nor the authors, contributors, or editors assume any liability for any injury and/or damage to persons or property as a matter of product's liability, negligence, or otherwise, or from any use or operation of any methods, products, instructions, or ideas contained in the material herein.

Content Strategist: Sandra Clark
Content Development Manager: Laurie Gower
Content Development Specialist: Heather Bays
Publishing Services Manager: Hemamalini Rajendrababu
Project Manager: Andrea Lynn Villamero

Printed in the United States of America

Last digit is the print number: 9   8   7   6   5   4   3   2   1

 Working together to grow libraries in developing countries

www.elsevier.com • www.bookaid.org

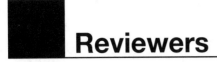

Reviewers

William T. Campbell, BSN, MS, Ed.D, RN
Associate Professor
Salisbury University
Salisbury, Maryland

Claire M. Creamer, PhD, RN, CPNP-PC
Assistant Professor of Nursing
RI College School of Nursing
Providence, Rhode Island

Christina D. Keller, MSN, RN, CHSE
Instructor
School of Nursing
Clinical Simulation Center
Radford University
Radford, Virginia

Denise Millot, MSN, RN
Clinical Facilities Coordinator/Senior Instructor – Pediatrics
Beth El College of Nursing and Health Sciences
Colorado Springs, Colorado

Patricia Munno, MSN, CPN, RN
Instructor for Nursing
Felician College
Lodi, New Jersey

Theresa Rhodes, MSN, RN
Instructor
Dishman Department of Nursing
Lamar University
Beaumont, Texas

Donna Wilsker, MSN, BSN, RN
Assistant Professor
Dishman Department of Nursing
Lamar University
Beaumont, Texas

Acknowledgments

We would like to acknowledge the editors and contributors for once again creating a comprehensive and informative nursing textbook, *Wong's Essentials of Pediatric Nursing,* Tenth Edition. In addition, we would like to thank the reviewers who offered constructive criticism and suggestions that added great merit to this workbook. Thank you, Elsevier, especially Sandra Clark and Heather Bays, for providing valuable support and assistance.

Best of all, we would like to thank our families for their patience and support during the update of this workbook. Kelley would like to thank her husband Jason and her three boys Levin (11 years old), Valen (8 years old), and Sajin (6 years old). Cheryl would like to thank her husband Eric. We are honored to be among the many talented nursing professionals at Elsevier working to improve the learning experience of student nurses.

Kelley Ward and Cheryl C. Rodgers

Contents

Chapter 1:   Perspectives of Pediatric Nursing   1

Chapter 2:   Community-Based Nursing Care of the Child and Family   7

Chapter 3:   Family Influences on Child Health Promotion   13

Chapter 4:   Communication and Physical Assessment of the Child and Family   19

Chapter 5:   Pain Assessment in Children   29

Chapter 6:   Infectious Disease   38

Chapter 7:   Health Promotion of the Newborn and Family   44

Chapter 8:   Health Problems of Newborns   56

Chapter 9:   Health Promotion of the Infant and Family   67

Chapter 10:   Health Problems of Infants   73

Chapter 11:   Health Promotion of the Toddler and Family   79

Chapter 12:   Health Promotion of the Preschooler and Family   87

Chapter 13:   Health Problems of Toddlers and Preschoolers   94

Chapter 14:   Health Promotion of the School-Age Child and Family   103

Chapter 15:   Health Promotion of the Adolescent and Family   109

Chapter 16:   Health Problems of School-Age Children and Adolescents   114

Chapter 17:   Quality of Life for Children Living with Chronic or Complex Diseases   124

Chapter 18:   Impact of Cognitive or Sensory Impairment on the Child and Family   133

Chapter 19:   Family Centered Care of the Child During Illness and Hospitalization   139

Chapter 20:   Pediatric Variations of Nursing Interventions   146

Chapter 21:   The Child with Respiratory Dysfunction   154

Chapter 22:   The Child with Gastrointestinal Dysfunction   168

Chapter 23:   The Child with Cardiovascular Dysfunction   179

Chapter 24:   The Child with Hematologic or Immunologic Dysfunction   188

Chapter 25:   The Child with Cancer   199

Chapter 26:   The Child with Genitourinary Dysfunction   207

Chapter 27:   The Child with Cerebral Dysfunction   214

Chapter 28:   The Child with Endocrine Dysfunction   227

Chapter 29:   The Child with Musculoskeletal or Articular Dysfunction   237

Chapter 30:   The Child with Neuromuscular or Muscular Dysfunction   247

Answer Key   254

1 Perspectives of Pediatric Nursing

Chapter 1 provides an overview of the nursing care of children from a child-centered perspective as unique individuals with specific developmental needs. The chapter explores the current state of health care for children, childhood health problems, and family-centered care. After completing this chapter, the student will be able to use the nursing process as a tool to critically think about ways to deliver individualized and effective nursing care to children and their families.

REVIEW OF ESSENTIAL CONCEPTS

Health Care for Children

1. Which of the following is the most common cause of death and disability to children aged 1 to 4 years in the United States?
   a. Fires and burns
   b. Firearms
   c. Unintentional injuries
   d. Falls

2. Which of the following best defines the primary goal of Healthy People 2020?
   a. Reduce substance and tobacco use through educative measures.
   b. Increase quality and length of life, and eliminate health disparities.
   c. Avoid injury and violence by adhering to preventive health outcomes.
   d. Provide access to care and immunizations to avoid potential injuries and health disparities.

3. The health status of children has improved in the past few years in a number of areas. Which best describes how the health status of children has improved?
   a. Average reading scores for fourth- through eighth-grade students have increased.
   b. The percentage of children living in poverty has decreased.
   c. The percentage of children with at least one parent employed full time year-round has decreased.
   d. The violent crime victimization rate among youth has decreased.

4. What is considered to be the most dramatic time of physical, motor, cognitive, emotional, and social development?
   a. Development that occurs during infancy
   b. Development that occurs during gestation
   c. Development that occurs during preschool
   d. Every stage of development in a child's life

5. Which of the following is the single most common chronic disease of childhood?
   a. Cancer
   b. Obesity
   c. Dental caries
   d. Otitis media

6. Children who grow up with an inadequate intake of nutritional foods are at risk for certain negative outcomes. Which of the following is the most recognized negative outcome related to inadequate nutrition?
   a. Infections and reading delays
   b. Appropriate protein intake with a reduction in sugar and carbohydrate intake
   c. Negative caloric intake with behavioral problems
   d. Growth and developmental delays and depression

Childhood Health Problems

7. Pediatric social illness is the new morbidity. Which statement best describes pediatric social illness?
   a. The behavior, social, and educational problems that children face
   b. The influence of culture and society in the health disparities of children
   c. The national health trend toward identifying and eliminating mental health problems in children
   d. Childhood illnesses that are a direct effect of the environment in which children live

1

8. You are observing a nurse who is caring for a 14-year-old boy in the pediatric clinic. Which of the following should you recognize to be the most common nutritional problem among American children?
   a. The 14-year-old boy has multiple dental caries.
   b. The 14-year-old boy's body mass index is at the 97th percentile for children of the same age.
   c. The 14-year-old boy reports consuming large amounts of sugar at each meal.
   d. The 14-year-old boy's height is in the 55th percentile for children of the same age.

Mortality

9. Which of the following has surpassed motor vehicle accidents as the leading cause of injury and mortality in children?
   a. Drowning
   b. Burns
   c. Head injuries
   d. Suicide

10. Define infant mortality.

11. Which of the following increases the risk of childhood suicide by about fivefold and the risk of homicide by about threefold?
    a. Exposure to violent video games
    b. Presence of a gun in a household
    c. Exposure to violence in the home
    d. Growing up in a disadvantaged neighborhood

12. Which of the following best describes the major determinant of neonatal death in technologically developed countries?
    a. Maternal education level
    b. Birth weight
    c. Amount of prenatal care
    d. Health care services

13. Which of the following is true with regard to African-American infants in the United States?
    a. They are at a lower risk of infant mortality compared with Caucasian infants.
    b. They are at a lower risk of low birth weight compared with Caucasian infants.
    c. Their infant mortality risk is two times higher than that of Caucasian infants.
    d. Their infant mortality risk is three times higher than that of Caucasian infants.

14. Identify the four most common causes of death during infancy.
    a.

    b.

    c.

    d.

15. Which age group has the lowest rate of death?
    a. Children aged 2 to 3 years
    b. Children aged 15 to 17 years
    c. Children aged 5 to 14 years
    d. Children aged 2 to 4 years

2

Morbidity

16. What is the chief illness of childhood?
    a. Bacterial infections
    b. Viral infections
    c. Meningitis
    d. Common cold

Philosophy of Care

17. Which of the following scenarios best describes how empowerment can be used to promote family-centered care?
    a. Creating opportunities and means for all family members to display their current abilities
    b. Providing the family with opportunities to acquire new abilities
    c. Providing care that meets the immediate needs of the family
    d. Providing an environment where the family has a sense of control over their lives by fostering their own strengths, abilities, and actions

Atraumatic Care

18. Atraumatic care is the provision of therapeutic care in settings, by personnel, and through the use of interventions

    that eliminate or minimize the _____ and _____ distress experienced by

    children and their families in the health care system.

19. List the three principles that provide the framework for achieving the goal in providing atraumatic care.
    a.

    b.

    c.

Role of the Pediatric Nurse

20. The establishment of a _____ is the essential foundation for providing high-quality nursing care.

21. Which of the following is a warning sign of a nontherapeutic relationship?
    a. Staff members voicing concerns about their peer's actions with a family
    b. Open communication between staff and family
    c. Staff offering anticipatory guidance before procedures
    d. Care provided to reduce or eliminate pain or discomfort

22. In a therapeutic relationship, caring, well-defined _____ separate the nurse from the child and family.

23. As an advocate, the nurse assists children and their families in making informed choices and acting in the child's best interests. Please choose the best answer from the statements below. Advocacy involves ensuring that families are
    a. aware of all available health services.
    b. informed and involved in treatments and procedures.
    c. encouraged to change or support existing health care practices.
    d. all of the above.

24. One of the most important aspects of providing pediatric care is that the care's focus is often on _____ measures.
    a. secondary
    b. preventative
    c. treatment
    d. remedy

25. Which of the following is often perceived by families as quality nursing care?
    a. Care focused on the technical needs of the child and family
    b. Care focused on the nontechnical needs of the child and family
    c. Care focused on the general needs of the child
    d. Care focused on the nursing process

26. Which of the following is the best approach to disease prevention?
    a. Quick and adequate treatment
    b. Family-centered care
    c. Education and anticipatory guidance
    d. Communication and building rapport

27. What is an indirect health-teaching strategy?
    a. Encouraging a parent to learn cardiopulmonary resuscitation
    b. Teaching a family how to bathe an infant
    c. Teaching a parent how to feed a newborn
    d. Encouraging parents to ask questions

28. When caring for a child, the nurse recognizes that the following intervention is the best way to facilitate nonverbal communication:
    a. Touching and physical presence
    b. Verbal communication
    c. Anticipatory guidance
    d. Play

29. Which of the following moral values is recognized as the obligation to minimize or prevent harm?
    a. Justice
    b. Nonmaleficence
    c. Beneficence
    d. Autonomy

30. The art of questioning why something is effective and whether a better approach exists is best described as
    a. intuition.
    b. the nursing process.
    c. evidence-based practice.
    d. problem solving.

Critical Thinking and the Process of Nursing Children and Families

31. Which of the following describes the GRADE criteria that indicate a high quality of evidence?
    a. Consistent evidence from well-performed randomized clinical trials (RCTs) or exceptionally strong evidence from unbiased observational studies
    b. Evidence from RCTs with important limitations (inconsistent results, flaws in methodology, indirect evidence, or imprecise results) or unusually strong evidence from unbiased observational studies
    c. Evidence for at least one critical outcome from observational studies, from RCTs with serious flaws, or from indirect evidence
    d. Evidence for at least one of the critical outcomes from unsystematic clinical observations or very indirect evidence

32. Describe clinical reasoning.

The Nursing Process

33. Define the nursing process, and list its five steps.

    a.

    b.

    c.

    d.

    e.

34. Match each of the following definitions with the appropriate term.

    a. _____ Assessment

    b. _____ Diagnosis

    c. _____ Planning

    d. _____ Implementation

    e. _____ Evaluation

    1. Once the nursing diagnoses have been identified, the nurse engages in this to establish outcomes or goals.
    2. This is a continuous process that operates at all phases of problem solving and is the foundation for decision making.
    3. This phase begins when the nurse puts the selected intervention into action and accumulates feedback data regarding its effects.
    4. This phase begins when the nurse must interpret and make decisions about the data gathered.
    5. In this phase the nurse gathers, sorts, and analyzes data to determine whether (1) the established outcome has been met, (2) the nursing interventions were appropriate, (3) the plan requires modification, or (4) other alternatives should be considered.

35. The three components of nursing diagnosis are _____, _____, and _____.

36. Match each of the following definitions with the appropriate term.

    a. _____ Problem statement

    b. _____ Etiology

    c. _____ Signs and symptoms

    1. Describes the child's response to health pattern deficits in the child, family, or community
    2. The cluster of cues and/or defining characteristics derived from the patient assessment
    3. The physiologic, situational, and maturational factors that cause the problem or influence its development

37. Define quality of care.

APPLYING CRITICAL THINKING TO NURSING PRACTICE

A. Spend a day following a nurse in a pediatric unit of an acute care facility. Briefly describe and give examples of the roles of the pediatric nurse in a pediatric unit.
   1. Family advocacy

2. Disease prevention and health promotion

3. Restorative role

4. Coordination and collaboration

5. Ethical decision making

6. Research

7. Family-centered care

B. You observe the care of a group of five children in an acute care unit of a children's hospital for one shift. Identify whether the principle of family-centered care is being applied or violated in the following examples. What steps could be taken to make these situations more family centered?
1. A child's father is allowed to visit for 3 hours a day. During his visitation time, the nurse decides to give the child a bath and asks the father to wait outside in the waiting room.

2. The posted visiting hours are noon to 8 pm for families, and no children under 14 years of age are allowed.

3. A mother changes the dressing on her child's leg. The nurse observes and assists as necessary.

4. The nurse would like to perform the morning bath on a child, but the nurse notes the child's mother is just awakening. The nurse asks the mother whether she would prefer the bath to occur now or at a time more convenient for her and the child.

6

2 Community-Based Nursing Care of the Child and Family

Chapter 2 explores the nurse's role in the multidisciplinary approach to the care of children and families in a community setting. Concepts and principles of community health nursing are studied. The components of the community nursing process are explained and contrasted with the nursing process used for an individual child or family. The information in this chapter will assist the student in defining and describing the community health nurse's different roles and functions in providing care for the child and family.

REVIEW OF ESSENTIAL CONCEPTS

Community Concepts

1. Which of the following definitions views the family from an economic standpoint?
   a. Interpersonal aspects of the family and its responsibility for personality development
   b. A productive unit providing for material needs.
   c. A social unit interacting with the larger society, creating the context within which cultural values and identity are formed
   d. Fulfilling the biologic function of perpetuation of the species

Family Theories

2. Which of the following theories is derived from general systems theory, a science of "wholeness" characterized by interaction among the components of the system and between the system and the environment?
   a. Family stress theory
   b. Developmental theory
   c. Family systems theory
   d. Resilience theory

3. What is one of the primary emphases of Bowen's family theory?
   a. Family members do not distinguish between one another emotionally or intellectually.
   b. The family unit has a high level of enmeshment and rigid control.
   c. When problems arise within the family, change occurs by maintaining the interaction or feedback messages that perpetuate disruptive behavior.
   d. Positive feedback initiates change, negative feedback resists change.

4. Which of the following predictable stressors are identified by the family stress theory?
   a. Divorce
   b. Illness
   c. Unemployment
   d. Parenthood

5. Which theory identifies the family as a small group (ie, a semiclosed system of personalities that interacts with the larger cultural social system)?
   a. Developmental theory
   b. Family systems theory
   c. Family stress theory
   d. Resilience theory

6. What is the most effective way for nurses to identify family strengths and weaknesses?
   a. Asking open-ended questions
   b. Observing for family patterns
   c. Performing a detailed nursing assessment
   d. Making assumptions based on past experience with families

7. Match each family structure with its description.

a. _____ Traditional nuclear family
b. _____ Blended family
c. _____ Single parent
d. _____ Binuclear family
e. _____ Polygamous family
f. _____ Communal family
g. _____ Gay, lesbian, bisexual, and transgender family

1. Family is one in which there is a legal or common-law tie between two persons of the same sex who have children
2. May have divergent beliefs, practices, and organization; the basic impetus for formation is often dissatisfaction with the nuclear family structure, social systems, and goals of the larger community
3. The conjugal unit is sometimes extended by the addition of spouses
4. Parents continuing the parenting role while terminating the spousal unit
5. Has emerged partially as a consequence of the women's rights movement and also as a result of more women (and men) establishing separate households because of divorce, death, or desertion
6. Also called a reconstituted family, includes at least one stepparent, stepsibling, or half-sibling
7. Composed of two parents and their children; the parent-child relationship may be biologic, step, adoptive, or foster

8. Which of the following is primarily responsible for shaping children's roles?
   a. Teachers
   b. Parents
   c. Siblings
   d. Friends

9. The nursing student observes a parent instructing her child to sit still by controlling the child's behavior through unquestioned mandates. She keeps telling her child to sit still "because I said so!" The nursing student recognizes this style of parenting to be
   a. permissive.
   b. authoritative.
   c. authoritarian.
   d. none of the above.

10. The parenting style that includes control that is firm and consistent but tempered with encouragement, understanding,

    and security is referred to as _____

    _____.

11. Which of the following is recognized to be a common cause for misbehavior in children?
    a. Desire for attention
    b. Feeling of acceptance
    c. Display of regression
    d. Display of adequacy

12. A school-age boy is stomping around at the clinic, dropping markers on the floor, and saying in an angry tone, "I can't make the picture look right!" The nursing student noticed that his mother said, "You are in so much trouble for acting this way. Just wait until I tell your father how bad you were at the doctor's office!" The nursing student recognizes this type of discipline is ineffective because
    a. the child's feelings are being maximized.
    b. the mother is delaying punishment.
    c. the father is not present.
    d. the child's behavior is normal and does not need to be addressed.

13. At what age is reasoning appropriate to use when addressing negative behavior in children?
    a. Infancy
    b. Preschool
    c. School age
    d. Toddlers

14. The best type of consequences of negative behavior in children is
    a. natural or logical.
    b. negative reinforcement.
    c. withdrawing privileges.
    d. grounding.

15. Which of the following discipline strategies by parents may interfere with the child's development and moral reasoning?
    a. Use of time-out
    b. Withdrawing privileges
    c. Corporal punishment
    d. Negative reinforcement

16. The nursing student is caring for an adopted preteen. Which of the following interventions is the most important to provide for the parents of this child?
    a. Reassuring their child that they understand the need to search for their identity.
    b. Planning for their child to reconnect with his or her biologic parents.
    c. Reminding their child that they have his or her best interest in mind.
    d. Tempering the child's desire to discover more information about his or her biologic parents.

17. Which of the following are common feelings 2- to 3-year-old children have when their parents are going through a divorce?
    a. Fear of abandonment
    b. Blaming themselves for the divorce; decreased self-esteem
    c. Bewilderment regarding all human relationships
    d. Fear and confusion

18. Which of the following are common feelings 9- to 12-year-old adolescents have when their parents are going through a divorce?
    a. Expression of anger, sadness, shame, and/or embarrassment
    b. Withdrawal from family and friends
    c. Disturbed concept of sexuality
    d. Decline in school performance

19. Which of the following social supports and community resources help meet the needs of single-parent families?
    a. Traditional health care services with typical office hours
    b. Respite child care to relieve parental exhaustion
    c. Promotion and acceptance of children taking on adult responsibilities
    d. Activities designed to increase the child's exposure to two-parent families

20. Define joint legal custody.

21. Indicate whether each of the following statements is true or false.
    a. **T F** When reprimanding children, focus only on the misbehavior, not on the child.
    b. **T F** Logical consequences occur without any intervention, such as being late and missing dinner.
    c. **T F** Consistency is when disciplinary action is implemented exactly as agreed on for each infraction.

22. Indicate whether each of the following statements is true or false.
    a. **T F** Children from lower-income, single-mother, and mother-partner families are considerably more likely to be living in foster care.
    b. **T F** Children in foster care are less likely to have a higher than normal incidence of acute and chronic health problems than children who are not in foster care.
    c. **T F** Foster children are often at risk because of their previous caretaking environment.

9

23. Which theorist states that a person's behavior results from the interaction of his or her traits and abilities with the environment?
    a. Piaget
    b. Maslow
    c. Bronfenbrenner
    d. Vygotsky

24. The nursing student recognizes that _____ is an important institution in which children systematically learn about the negative consequences of behavior that departs from social expectations.
    a. church
    b. athletics
    c. school
    d. family

25. Describe four categories of external assets that youth receive from the community.
    a. Support
    b. Empowerment
    c. Boundaries and expectations
    d. Constructive use of time

APPLYING CRITICAL THINKING TO THE NURSING PRACTICE

A. Interview an expectant couple and then parents with a school-age child to contrast their views of parenthood. Answer the following questions. Include the parents' responses to illustrate these concepts.
   1. According to Duvall's developmental stages of the family theory, what are the tasks for each of the following families? Are the families you interviewed successful in accomplishing these tasks?
       a. Expectant couple

       b. Parents of a school-age child

   2. What factors affect the transition to parenthood?

B. After talking with a variety of families with children of various developmental ages, answer the following questions that deal with the effects of different family structures on child development. Include specific examples to illustrate these concepts.
   1. What life events might alter family structure?

   2. What implication does an alteration in composition have for the family and child?

   3. List the qualities of strong families, regardless of their configuration.
       a.

b.

c.

d.

e.

f.

g.

h.

i.

j.

k.

l.

C. Talk to a working, recently divorced single parent to assess problem areas. Answer the following questions.
 1. What changes or feelings accompany single parenthood?

 2. List four social supports and community resources needed by single-parent families.
  a.

  b.

  c.

  d.

D. Interview a couple who consist of dual-career parents and a couple who consist of a stay-at-home parent and a career parent. Assess both problem and strength areas in these families. Identify two strengths and two weaknesses associated with the dual-career parents and with the stay-at-home parent and career parent.

3 Family Influences on Child Health Promotion

Chapter 3 provides an overview of family and parenting influences on the health promotion of children. Different family structures, functions, and roles are explored. Motivation, preparation, and transition to parenting are presented and discussed. After completing this chapter, the student will have information on a variety of family situations that will form a foundation for developing appropriate nursing strategies to promote the health of children.

REVIEW OF ESSENTIAL CONCEPTS

Growth and Development

1. Match each term with its definition.

   a. _____ Growth

   b. _____ Maturation

   c. _____ Development

   d. _____ Differentiation

   1. An increase in competence, adaptability, and aging, usually used to describe a qualitative change; a change in the complexity of a structure that makes it possible for that structure to begin functioning; to function at a higher level
   2. A gradual growth and expansion involving a change from lower to more advanced stages of complexity
   3. An increase in the number and size of cells as they divide and synthesize new proteins; results in increased size and weight of the whole or any of its parts
   4. A biologic description of the processes by which early cells and structures are modified and altered to achieve specific, characteristic physical and chemical properties

2. Growth can be viewed as a(n) _____ change, and development as a(n) _____ change.

3. Which of the following best characterizes the patterns of human growth and development?
   a. Continuous and common
   b. Unpredictable and orderly
   c. Predictable and regressive
   d. Continuous and predictable

4. Which of the following describes a set of skills and competencies peculiar to each developmental stage that children must accomplish or master in order to deal effectively with their environment?
   a. Growth
   b. Developmental task
   c. Regression
   d. Maturation

5. Define and describe cephalocaudal development.

6. Define and describe proximodistal development.

7. Generalized development precedes specific or specialized development. _____ movements take place before _____ muscle control.

8. Indicate whether each of the following statements is true or false.
   a. **T   F**   In growth and development, there is a definite, predictable sequence with each child normally passing through every stage.
   b. **T   F**   Growth and development progress at the same pace and rate in all humans.
   c. **T   F**   The last 3 months of prenatal life are the most sensitive periods for physical growth of the fetus.

9. For each of the following stages of development, match the body part in which growth predominates.
   a. _____ Prenatal
   b. _____ Infancy
   c. _____ Early and middle childhood
   d. _____ Adolescence

   1. Trunk predominates
   2. Head
   3. Trunk elongates
   4. Legs

10. At what age does one double the child's height to estimate how tall he or she will be as an adult?
    a. 1 year
    b. 2 years
    c. 18 months
    d. 8 months

11. By _____ to _____ months of age, the birth weight doubles. By the end of the

    first year, it _____. By age 2, the birth weight usually _____.

12. Which of the following is recognized as the most accurate measure of general development?
    a. Height
    b. Muscle mass
    c. Bone age
    d. Weight-to-height ratio

13. Which of the following factors does not influence skeletal muscle injury rates and types in children and adolescents?
    a. Improper or inadequate use of protective sports equipment for children
    b. Inadequate conditioning, especially in flexibility
    c. The rapid growth rate of the epiphyseal zone of hypertrophy in adolescents
    d. Neuromuscular development at various stages of development

Development of Organ Systems

14. Describe the process of lymphoid tissue development in humans.

15. What determines the caloric requirements of children?

16. What is the basal energy requirement of infants?
    a. About 108 kcal/kg of body weight
    b. About 110 kcal/kg of body weight
    c. About 109 kcal/kg of body weight
    d. About 111 kcal/kg of body weight

17. In the healthy neonate, what three negative metabolic consequences can occur as a result of hypothermia?
    a.

    b.

    c.

18. The length of a sleep cycle increases from approximately 50 to 60 minutes in the newborn infant to approximately

_____ minutes in adolescence.

19. Identify the temperamental category described by each of the following.
    a. Highly active, irritable, and irregular in habits, such as feeding and sleep; adapts slowly to routines, people, and new situations
    b. Reacts negatively and mildly intensely to new stimuli and situations; is inactive and moody but shows only moderate irregularity in functions
    c. Even-tempered, regular, and predictable in habits; has a positive approach to new stimuli and situations; is open and adaptable to change

20. Children who display the difficult or slow-to-warm-up patterns of behavior are more vulnerable to the development

of _____ in early and middle childhood.

Development of Personality and Mental Function

21. Match the five stages of psychosexual development (Freud) with the ages encompassed by each.

    a. _____ Oral stage
    b. _____ Anal stage
    c. _____ Latency period
    d. _____ Genital stage
    e. _____ Phallic stage

    1. 1 to 3 years
    2. Birth to 1 year
    3. 3 to 6 years
    4. 6 to 12 years
    5. 12 to 18 years

22. For each of the following age groups, identify Erikson's stage of psychosocial development.
    a. Birth to 1 year
    b. 1 to 3 years
    c. 3 to 6 years
    d. 6 to 12 years
    e. 12 to 18 years

23. Match each stage of cognitive development (Piaget) with its defining characteristics (more than one answer may apply).

    a. _____ Sensorimotor stage (birth to 2 years)
    b. _____ Preoperational stage (2 to 7 years)
    c. _____ Concrete operations (7 to 11 years)
    d. _____ Formal operations (11 to 15 years)

    1. Predominant characteristic is egocentrism.
    2. Thought is adaptable and flexible.
    3. Child progresses from reflex activity to imitative behavior; problem solving is trial and error.
    4. Thought becomes increasingly logical and coherent; conservation is developed; problems are solved in a concrete, systematic fashion.
    5. Child displays a high level of curiosity, experimentation, and enjoyment of novelty and begins to develop a sense of self as he or she is able to differentiate the self from the environment.
    6. Child can think in abstract terms, use abstract symbols, and draw logical conclusions from a set of operations.
    7. Child can now consider a point of view other than his or her own; socialized thinking occurs.
    8. Child is unable to see things from any perspective other than his or her own; thinking is concrete.

24. What factors contribute to the rate of speech development?
    a. Neurologic competence and cognitive development
    b. Musculoskeletal competence and cognitive development
    c. Social factors and neurologic competence
    d. Hereditary factors and cognitive development

25. At all stages of language development, a child's _____ vocabulary is greater than his or her

_____ vocabulary.

26. Describe the three stages of moral development (Kohlberg).
   a. Preconventional morality
   b. Conventional level
   c. Postconventional, autonomous, or principled level

Development of Self-Concept

27. Define *self-concept*.

28. Self-concept at _____ is described as an awareness of one's independent existence learned in part as a result of social contacts and experiences with others.
   a. Infancy
   b. Toddlerhood
   c. School age
   d. Adolescence

29. Which of the following is described as the subjective concepts and attitudes that individuals have toward their own bodies?
   a. Self-concept
   b. Body image
   c. Self-knowledge
   d. Self-esteem

30. _____, or the value that an individual places on himself or herself, refers to an overall evaluation of oneself.

Role of Play in Development

31. Match each type of play with its defining characteristics.

   a. _____ Solitary play

   b. _____ Cooperative play

   c. _____ Onlooker play

   d. _____ Associative play

   e. _____ Parallel play

   1. Child watches what other children are doing but makes no attempt to enter into the play activity. An example is watching an older sibling color a picture.
   2. Child plays alone and independently with toys different from those of other children within the same area. The child's interest is centered on his or her own activity.
   3. Child plays independently among other children with toys that are like those that the children around him or her are using, neither influencing nor being influenced by them. There is no group association.
   4. Child plays with other children, engaging in a similar or identical activity in which there is no organization, division of labor, or mutual goal. An example is two children playing with dolls.
   5. Child plays in a group with other children with discussion and planning of activities for accomplishing an end.

32. List the seven functions that play serves to develop throughout childhood.
   a.

   b.

   c.

d.

e.

f.

g.

33. Research has indicated that a positive _____ interaction can enhance early childhood brain development.

Selected Factors That Influence Development

34. The _____ developmental screening test is no longer recommended by the American Academy of Neurology or the Child Neurology Society.

35. Which of the following is the single most important influence on growth?
   a. Hereditary
   b. Activity level
   c. Nutrition
   d. Musculoskeletal development

36. The _____ is unquestionably the single most influential person during early infancy.

37. Which term is used to refer to a particular form of a gene?
   a. Sites
   b. Loci
   c. Allele
   d. Gene

38. Abnormal formations of organs or body parts resulting from an abnormal developmental process are referred to as
   a. disruptions.
   b. congenital malformations.
   c. dysplasias.
   d. malformations.

APPLYING CRITICAL THINKING TO THE NURSING PRACTICE

A. Levi, a 1-year-old boy, comes into the clinic for a well-child visit. The nurse assesses Levi's growth and development. Interpret the following assessment data.
   1. Levi weighed 3.2 kg (7 pounds, 2 ounces) at birth. His weight today is 10 kg (22 pounds). Is this a normal increase? If not, what would be the expected gain?

   2. Levi's mother wants to know whether his height at this age has any significance for his adult height. What should the nurse tell her?

Chapter **3** **Family Influences on Child Health Promotion**

3. The nurse observes Levi interacting with his mother. After the assessment, Levi wants to be held closely by his mother. His mother gladly pulls him into her body. Describe Levi's mother's response to him.

B. Observe a child from each age group: infant, toddler, preschool, school age, and adolescent.
   1. Although children vary in both their rate of growth and their acquisition of developmental skills, certain predictable patterns are universal and basic to all human beings. Why is this factor important for nurses to understand?

   2. Identify the psychosocial conflict of each age group, provide a specific intervention that will assist in the resolution of this conflict, and describe the unfavorable conflict (Erikson).
      a. Infant

      b. Toddler

      c. Preschool

      d. School age

      e. Adolescent
   3. Describe the characteristics of spiritual development in each age group.
      a. Infant

      b. Toddler

      c. Preschool

      d. School age

      e. Adolescent

C. Interview the parents of a newborn regarding the infant's temperament.
   1. Why is it important to assess a child's temperament?

   2. List behaviors typical of the following temperament patterns.
      a. The easy child
      b. The difficult child

4 Communication and Physical Assessment of the Child and Family

Chapter 4 introduces the essential components of communication and physical assessment in the nursing care of children. Communication, along with physical and developmental assessment, is an essential skill of nurses who care for children and their families. Guidelines for effectively communicating, taking a health history, and performing a physical assessment are presented. At the completion of this chapter, the student will have the foundation to assess communication patterns and the child's physical and developmental progress.

REVIEW OF ESSENTIAL CONCEPTS

Guidelines for Communicating and Interviewing

1. When the nurse is interviewing a child and his or her family, which three characteristics of the physical environment in which the interview occurs contribute to an effective interview?

   a.

   b.

   c.

2. What information obtained during an interview cannot be kept confidential?
   a. Reports of consensual sexual activity
   b. Suicidal ideation
   c. Peer pressure
   d. Drug use

3. What are successful outcomes of triage services based on?
   a. Accuracy and consistency of data provided
   b. Timing of the call
   c. Education of the triage nurse
   d. The latest technological advances

Communicating with Families

4. Which approach is used to direct the focus of the interview while allowing maximum freedom of expression?
   a. Asking open-ended questions
   b. Having the parent fill out a questionnaire
   c. Asking the parent to choose from a list of possible answers
   d. Asking the parent to paint a picture of a typical day in the child's life

5. What is the most important component of effective communication?
   a. Talking
   b. Silence
   c. Listening
   d. Understanding

6. Which of the following is an example of anticipatory guidance?
   a. The nurse changing a dressing before surgery
   b. The nurse preparing the child and parent for an upcoming procedure
   c. The nurse performing a head-to-toe assessment
   d. The nurse researching an effective way to meet a patient outcome.

19

7. Identify three signs of information overload.

   a.

   b.

   c.

8. What is an important factor to recognize when obtaining informed consent from an interpreter?
   a. The child or adolescent may not feel comfortable disclosing confidential information to the interpreter.
   b. The interpreter can be liable for damages if the child or parent failed to understand the procedure before giving consent.
   c. As long as the family understands the basics of the procedure, informed consent can be obtained.
   d. The nurse must fully inform the family of all aspects of the procedure before obtaining informed consent.

9. Indicate whether each of the following statements regarding interpreters is true or false.
   a. **T F** Communicate directly with the interpreter when asking questions to be as clear as possible.
   b. **T F** Limit the use of medical terms as much as possible.
   c. **T F** In obtaining informed consent through an interpreter, it is important that the family be fully informed of all aspects of the particular procedure to which they are consenting.
   d. **T F** When a child is translating, it is important to stress the need for literal translation of parent responses.

10. Match each communication strategy to the age group with which it is best used.

   a. _____ Infants
   b. _____ Young children
   c. _____ School-age children
   d. _____ Adolescents

   1. Tell them what they will do and how they will feel. Allow them to touch articles that will come in contact with them.
   2. Cuddle, pat, or gently hold them.
   3. Tell them what is going on and why it is being done to them. Explain all procedures to them in a specific manner.
   4. Be attentive and do not pry.

11. Which of the following is correct when assessing an adolescent's sexual health history?
   a. The nurse should start with the sexual health history before obtaining information on the adolescent's general health.
   b. The nurse should build a rapport with the adolescent before obtaining an adolescent's sexual health history.
   c. The nurse should refrain from asking an adolescent about his or her sexual health.
   d. The adolescent must have his or her parents present during the sexual health history part of the assessment.

Communication Techniques

12. _____ is the universal language of children.

13. How do play sessions serve the child and the nurse?
   a. They can be used as assessment tools.
   b. They can be used to determine the child's awareness of his or her illness.
   c. They can be used to determine the child's perception of his or her illness.
   d. All of the above.

History Taking

14. The _____ is the specific reason for the child's visit to the clinic, office, or hospital.

15. What is a narrative of the chief complaint from its earliest onset through its progression to the present?
   a. Present illness
   b. Health history
   c. Review of symptoms
   d. Documentation record

16. What is important to ask parents about when obtaining an immunization history?
    a. The names of the specific diseases immunized against
    b. The number of injections and if the child had any previous reactions
    c. The dosage and date when administered
    d. All of the above

17. Which of the following is the best question the nurse can ask to initiate a conversation about sexual concerns?
    a. "Tell me about your social life."
    b. "What are you learning about in school?"
    c. "Do you have a lot of friends?"
    d. "Do your friends have sex?"

18. What are the most important previous growth patterns to record?
    a.

    b.

    c.

19. The sexual history is an essential component of adolescents' health assessment. What are three important reasons for obtaining a sexual history?
    a.

    b.

    c.

Review of Systems

20. What is the primary purpose of the family medical history?
    a. To discover family communication patterns
    b. To discover hereditary and familial diseases
    c. To observe family roles and relationships
    d. To document family structure

21. What is the most common method of eliciting information on the family structure?
    a. Assessment
    b. Interview
    c. Interpretation
    d. Communication

22. Give an example of a broad statement with which the nurse can introduce the review of a specific system.

Nutritional Assessment

23. Match each dietary reference intake (DRI), or the four nutrient-based reference values, to the statement that describes it.

a. _____ Estimated average requirement (EAR)

b. _____ Recommended dietary allowance (RDA)

c. _____ Adequate intake (AI)

d. _____ Tolerable upper intake level (UL)

1. Average daily dietary intake sufficient to meet the nutrient requirement of nearly all (97 to 98%) healthy individuals for a specific age and gender group
2. Recommended intake level based on estimates of nutrient intake by healthy groups of individuals
3. Nutrient intake estimated to meet the requirement of half of the healthy individuals (50%) for a specific age and gender group
4. As intake increases above the UL, risk of adverse effects increase

24. What is the most common and probably easiest method of assessing daily intake?
    a. 24-Hour intake
    b. Food diary
    c. 3-Day intake
    d. Observation

CLINICAL EXAMINATION

25. _____, an essential parameter of nutritional status, is the measurement of height, weight, head circumference, proportions, skinfold thickness, and arm circumference in children.

Evaluation of Nutritional Assessment

26. What three conclusions can be drawn from the nutritional assessment data?
    a.

    b.

    c.

General Approaches to Examining the Child

27. What are the most common laboratory studies to assess children for undernutrition?
    a. Hemoglobin, red blood cell indices, and serum albumin or prealbumin
    b. Liver enzymes, red blood cell indices, and serum albumin or prealbumin
    c. Lipids, red blood cell indices, and serum albumin or prealbumin
    d. Fasting serum glucose, red blood cell indices, and serum albumin or prealbumin

Physical Examination

28. Weight, height (length), skinfold thickness, arm circumference, and head circumference are

    _____.

29. The most prominent change to the complement of growth charts for older children and adolescents is the addition of

    the _____ growth curves.

30. Why is it essential that nurses understand the revised growth charts?

31. Which of the following may indicate questionable growth in a child?
    a. Both parents and child have short stature
    b. Height and weight percentiles are similar
    c. Showing steady patterns of growth
    d. Failure to follow the expected growth velocity in height and weight, especially during the rapid growth periods of infancy and adolescence

32. Measurements taken when a child is supine are referred to as _____, whereas measurements taken when the child is standing upright are referred to as _____.

33. What is an important safety measure to take when measuring an infant's weight?

34. One convenient measure of body fat is _____, which is measured with skin calipers.

35. Head circumference is measured in children up to _____ months of age.

Physiologic Measurements

36. For best results in taking vital signs of infants, count _____ first (before the infant is disturbed), take the _____ next, and measure _____ last.

37. What is an acceptable rectal temperature in children?

38. What factor most affects the accuracy of temperature measurement?

39. Which site is best for assessing the pulse in infants? _____ Which site is best for assessing the pulse in children older than 2 years of age? _____

40. Are respirations in infants assessed by observing for diaphragmatic or intercostal breathing patterns?

41. What is the most important factor in ensuring a reliable blood pressure measurement?

Chapter **4** **Communication and Physical Assessment of the Child and Family**

42. Identify at least five causes of orthostatic hypotension in children.

   a.

   b.

   c.

   d.

   e.

43. If respirations in the infant are irregular, they should be counted for _____.

44. An accurate pulse in infants must be taken _____ for 1 full minute.

General Appearance

45. Match each abnormal color change with its description.

   a. _____ Cyanosis   1. Small pinpoint hemorrhages
                                   2. Blue tinge to the skin
   b. _____ Erythema   3. Redness of the skin
                                   4. Yellow staining of the skin
   c. _____ Jaundice

   d. _____ Petechiae

46. What two methods of assessment are primarily used to assess the skin?

   a.

   b.

47. What is a sign of poor nutrition?
   a. Hair that is stringy, dull, brittle, dry, friable, and depigmented
   b. Skin turgor less than 3 seconds
   c. Sweating after minimal exercise
   d. Hair that is shiny but thin

48. Describe the technique for palpating lymph nodes.

49. What is a serious sign of meningeal irritation?
   a. Stiff back
   b. Inability to lay on the left side
   c. Hyperextension of the head with pain on extension
   d. Hyperextension of the head with pain on flexion

50. Normal findings of examination of the pupils can be documented as _____.

51. The nurse can prepare the child for the ophthalmoscopic examination by doing the following three things.

    a.

    b.

    c.

52. The most common test for measuring visual acuity is the _____ letter chart.

53. Low-set ears are commonly associated with _____ or _____.

54. In infants and children younger than 3 years, assess the inner ear by pulling the pinna _____ and _____. In children older than 3 years, assess the inner ear by pulling the pinna _____ and _____.

55. What is the color of a normal tympanic membrane?

56. What is the reason for leaving assessment of the mouth toward the end of the physical assessment in children?

57. What is the respiratory movement typically observed in girls over age 7?
    a. Diaphragmatic
    b. Thoracic

Lung

58. Identify the three classifications or descriptions of lung sounds.

    a.

    b.

    c.

59. The two classifications of adventitious breath sounds are _____ and _____.

60. The apical impulse (AI) is found just lateral to the left midclavicular line and fourth intercostal space in children

_____ years of age and at the left midclavicular line and fifth intercostal space in children

_____ years of age.

61. To distinguish between S_1 and S_2 heart sounds, simultaneously palpate the carotid pulse with the index and middle

fingers and listen to the heart sounds. _____ is synchronous with the carotid pulse.

62. Identify and define the four characteristics for which heart sounds are evaluated.
    a.

    b.

    c.

    d.

63. When documenting a murmur, what four elements need to be recorded?
    a.

    b.

    c.

    d.

64. Indicate whether each of the following statements is true or false.
    a. **T** **F** The correct sequence for assessing the abdomen is inspection, palpation, and auscultation.
    b. **T** **F** A tense, boardlike abdomen is a serious sign of paralytic ileus and intestinal obstruction.
    c. **T** **F** A femoral hernia occurs more frequently in boys.
    d. **T** **F** Absence of femoral pulses is a significant sign of coarctation of the aorta and is referred for medical
         evaluation.

65. What approach should the nurse take when examining the genitalia of a child or adolescent?

66. A lateral curvature of the spine is called _____.

67. What is the most common gait problem in young children? What does it result from?

68. An estimation of muscle strength is assessed by having the child use an extremity to _____

 or _____ against resistance.

Neurologic Assessment

69. The _____ assessment is the broadest and most diverse part of the examining process.

70. To prevent younger children from _____ during the reflex assessment, the nurse should distract them with toys or talk to them.

APPLYING CRITICAL THINKING TO THE NURSING PRACTICE

A. Interview a preschool child and his or her family.
 1. What are the key elements of an appropriate introduction to an interview?

 2. Why is it important to include the parents in the problem-solving process?

 3. Identify one way to direct the focus of the interview while also allowing for maximum freedom of expression for both the family and child.

 4. What creative communication techniques are effective in encouraging communication with the child?

B. Mrs. Gonzales brings her son Val, age 3 months, to the pediatric clinic for an annual checkup. It is the first time they have visited the clinic. Mrs. Gonzales's English is poor. The Gonzales family has been living in the United States for 3 months.
 1. Identify at least four verbal strategies that would enhance the cultural sensitivity of the interaction.
  a.

  b.

  c.

  d.

2. During the interview, Mrs. Gonzales begins to comment about her two other children. What is an effective yet respectful way the nurse can redirect the focus of the interview?

3. What portion of the past history section of the health history is of particular importance because Val has been in this country only 3 months?

4. What additional information in the family medical history section of the health history would be important for the nurse to obtain from Mrs. Gonzales?

C. Todd, age 5 years, was referred to the nutrition clinic by the nurse practitioner. The nurse was concerned because Todd's weight was above the 90th percentile for his age. A complete nutritional assessment was performed.
   1. What three methods can Todd's mother use to record his dietary intake?
      a.

      b.

      c.

   2. Anthropometry is an important part of Todd's nutritional assessment. Why is it important?

   3. The results of the nutritional assessment reveal that Todd's mother knows little about nutrition, there is a history of overeating in Todd's family, and Todd's obesity is the result of his excessive intake of nutrients. Form two nursing diagnoses based on the assessment results.
      a.

      b.

D. Tina, age 4 years, is at urgent care because she is complaining of a sudden onset of abdominal pain.
   1. What are some ways the nurse can help Tina relax during the abdominal assessment?

   2. How can the nurse minimize the sensation of tickling during the examination?

5 Pain Assessment in Children

Chapter 5 provides the theoretical basis for assessing and managing pain in children. The chapter addresses pain in specific populations, including children in a variety of different cultures who have cognitive impairment or chronic illness. On completion of this chapter, the student will have the foundation to assess and manage pain in children.

REVIEW OF ESSENTIAL CONCEPTS

Pain Assessment

1. What is the purpose of a pediatric pain assessment?
   a. To determine how much pain the child is feeling
   b. To determine the dosage of pain medicine the child needs
   c. To evaluate whether the current pain medication regimen is working
   d. To rate the child's pain level

2. Which pain assessment method is useful for measuring pain in infants and preverbal children who do not have the language skills to communicate that they are in pain?

3. In what situations are behavioral measures most reliable when measuring pain?

4. What is a major disadvantage in using physiologic assessments for pain?

5. At what age are most children able to discriminate degrees of pain in facial expressions?
   a. By age 5
   b. By age 2
   c. By age 3
   d. By age 4

6. At what age can most children effectively use the 0 to 10 numeric rating scale that is currently used by adolescents and adults?
   a. From 7 to 10 years old
   b. From 5 to 7 years old
   c. From 6 to 8 years old
   d. From 8 to 10 years old

Pain Assessment in Specific Populations

7. Which of the following pain assessment tools is a ten point scale similar to the APGAR score?
   a. CRIES
   b. Adolescent Pediatric Pain Tool
   c. Pediatric Pain Questionnaire
   d. Neonatal Pain, Agitation, and Sedation Scale

Children with Communication and Cognitive Impairment

8. Which of the following pain scales is used to assess pain in children with cognitive impairment?
   a. Pediatric Pain Questionnaire (PPQ)
   b. CRIES
   c. Neonatal Pain, Agitation, and Sedation Scale (NPASS)
   d. Face, Legs, Activity, Cry, Consolability (FLACC)

9. Which of the following does the nurse recognize to be the most important source of information during a child's assessment?
   a. Primary caregiver
   b. Medical record
   c. Child's statements
   d. Extended family members

Cultural Issues in Pain Assessment

10. What does the nurse recognize to be a major challenge in the assessment and management of pain in children from different cultures?
    a. There is not a lot of difference among children of different cultures regarding pain assessment and management.
    b. The cultural appropriateness of pain assessment tools have been validated only in Caucasian and English-speaking children.
    c. The cultural appropriateness of pain assessment tools has been validated in a variety of cultures.
    d. The differences among children of different cultures regarding pain assessment and management are not important to managing pain in children.

11. Self-report observational scales and interview questionnaires for pain may not be a reliable measure of pain

    assessment in _____ children.
    a. Caucasian
    b. Native American
    c. Hispanic
    d. Asian

12. Which pain scale for children has been developed for use with Caucasian, African American, and Hispanic populations?

Children with Chronic Illness and Complex Pain

13. What is the most important factor during assessment of children with chronic illness, particularly during assessment of complex pain?

Pain Management

14. List at least four nonpharmacologic techniques that reduce pain perception in children.

    a.

    b.

    c.

    d.

15. Which of the following interventions have been demonstrated to have a calming and pain-relieving effect for invasive procedures in neonates?
    a. Loosening the infant's swaddling blanket to allow the infant to move freely
    b. Placing the infant in side-lying position
    c. Brightening the lights around the infant so the infant can observe his or her surroundings
    d. The administration of concentrated sucrose with and without nonnutritive sucking

16. Identify four benefits of infants who spend 1 to 3 hours in kangaroo care.

    a.

    b.

    c.

    d.

Complementary Pain Medicine

17. The following are five classifications of complementary and alternative medicine (CAM) therapies. Give some examples of each.
    a. Biologically based
    b. Manipulative treatments
    c. Energy based
    d. Mind-body techniques
    e. Alternative medical systems

Pharmacologic Management

18. What medications are suitable for mild to moderate pain in children?

19. What class of medications is used for severe pain in children?

20. What is the difference between nonopioids and opioids?
    a. Nonopioids primarily act at the central nervous system, and opioids primarily act at the peripheral nervous system.
    b. Nonopioids primarily act at the peripheral nervous system, and opioids primarily act at the central nervous system.
    c. There is not much of a difference between the action of nonopioids and opioids.
    d. Nonopioids are considered to be a nonpharmacologic method of pain management, while opioids are considered to be a pharmacologic method of pain management.

21. _____ is considered the gold standard for the management of severe pain.

22. Match each of the following adjuvants to the correct statement.

    a. _____ Tricyclic antidepressants

    b. _____ Antiepileptics

    c. _____ Stool softeners and laxatives

    d. _____ Antiemetics

    e. _____ Antianxiety

    f. _____ Diphenhydramine

    g. _____ Steroids

    h. _____ Dextroamphetamine and caffeine

    1. Senna and docusate sodium
    2. Gabapentin, carbamazepine, clonazepam
    3. Amitriptyline, imipramine
    4. Diazepam, midazolam
    5. Promethazine, droperidol
    6. For inflammation and pain
    7. Consider opioid switch if sedation is persistent
    8. For itching

23. Describe how the nurse determines the optimum dosage of an analgesic.

24. Indicate whether each of the following statements is true or false.
    a. **T F** Children (except infants younger than about 3 to 6 months) metabolize drugs less rapidly than adults do.
    b. **T F** Younger children may require higher doses of opioids to achieve the same analgesic effect.
    c. **T F** Children's dosages are usually calculated according to body weight, except in children with a weight greater than 50 kg (110 pounds), where use of the weight formula may mean that the children's dosage exceeds the average adult dosage.

25. Define a *ceiling effect*. Describe the major difference between opioids and nonopioids regarding a ceiling effect.

26. What are the requirements for a child to use a patient-controlled anesthesia (PCA) pump?

27. Which of the following is a typical case in which PCA is used for controlling pain?
    a. Surgery
    b. Sickle cell crisis
    c. Trauma
    d. All of the above

28. _____ is the drug of choice for PCA and is usually prepared in a concentration of 1 mg/mL.

29. PCA infusion devices typically allow for the following three methods or modes of drug administration to be used alone or in combination.
    a.

    b.

    c.

30. Match each of the following statements to the correct description.
    a. _____ Epidural analgesia

    b. _____ Intradermal analgesia

    c. _____ Transdermal analgesia

    1. LMX, fentanyl, EMLA, and LidoSite are examples of medications administered by this route.
    2. This route is used to inject a local anesthetic, typically lidocaine, into the skin to reduce the pain from a lumbar puncture, bone marrow aspiration, or venous or arterial access.
    3. A catheter is placed into a space of the spinal column at the lumbar or caudal level.

31. What is the most common reason for the mismanagement of infant pain?
    a. The medications available are not potent enough to manage infant pain.
    b. The medications available are designed for adults not infants.
    c. There are misconceptions regarding the effects of pain on the neonate.
    d. The dosage routes are mostly ineffective in infants.

32. Indicate whether each of the following statements is true or false.
    a. **T F** Preventive pain control is best provided through continuous intravenous (IV) infusion rather than intermittent boluses.
    b. **T F** The intervals between doses should exceed the drug's expected duration of effectiveness.
    c. **T F** Continuous analgesia is always appropriate in pain control of children.
    d. **T F** Respiratory depression is the most serious complication of analgesia and is most likely to occur in sedated patients.
    e. **T F** Lower limits of normal respiratory rates are not established for children.
    f. **T F** A slower respiratory rate does not necessarily reflect decreased arterial oxygenation.

33. Which of the following is a common, and sometimes serious, side effect of opioids?
    a. Urinary retention
    b. Hypertension
    c. Constipation
    d. Dry mouth

34. What two things can occur with prolonged use of opioids?

a.

b.

35. Describe the manifestations of the following symptoms of opioid withdrawal.

a. Neurologic excitability

b. Gastrointestinal dysfunction

c. Autonomic dysfunction

36. Which of the following patients should be weaned from opioids?
a. The neonate whose mother received opioids during labor and delivery
b. The infant who was administered opioids for 8 days
c. The infant who was administered opioids for 4 days
d. The neonate who received 24 hours of opioids

37. _____ occurs when the dose of an opioid needs to be increased to achieve the same analgesic effect previously achieved at a lower dose.

38. Explain whether infants or children can become psychologically dependent on or addicted to pain medication.

39. What tools are used to evaluate the effectiveness of pain regimens?

40. An infant was started on a pain management plan. When should the nurse evaluate the infant's response to drug therapy?
a. Immediately after treatment is commenced
b. 15 to 30 minutes after each dose is given
c. 30 to 45 minutes after each dose is given
d. Every 6 hours

41. Which of the following is a priority guiding principle of pain management?
a. Prevention of pain is always better than treatment
b. Treating pain levels rated at 5 and above
c. Providing nonpharmacologic pain relief measures before pharmacologic measures
d. Pain is a subjective experience

Painful and Invasive Procedures

42. Match each of the following statements with the correct response.

    a. _____ Caudal or penile blocks are used for

    b. _____ Bupivacaine is used for

    c. _____ Foam dressing soaked with bupivacaine is used for

    d. _____ A local anesthetic infiltration with bupivacaine is used for

    e. _____ Nitrous oxide inhalations are used for

1. open wounds.
2. circumcision pain.
3. minor and some intermediate procedures.
4. graft donor sites.
5. suture removal or dressing changes.

Postoperative Pain

43. Which four outcomes can be a result of severe postoperative pain due to sympathetic overactivity?

    a.

    b.

    c.

    d.

44. Which of the following techniques can help a burn patient relax and gain a sense of control?
    a. Hyponosis
    b. Relaxation training
    c. Psychotherapy
    d. All of the above

Recurrent Headaches in Children

45. What is the most disturbing symptom in migraine headaches?

46. Which of the following is the best method for obtaining assessment data on headaches in children?
    a. Rating
    b. Observing
    c. Headache diary
    d. Biofeedback

47. What are the two main behavioral approaches for preventing headaches in children?
    a.

    b.

Recurrent Abdominal Pain in Children

48. Define recurrent abdominal pain (RAP) in children.

35

49. The use of _____ therapy has been documented to reduce or eliminate pain in children with RAP and highlights the involvement of parents in supporting their child's self-management behavior.

Cancer Pain in Children

50. In young adult survivors of childhood cancer, _____ conditions may develop.

51. What are almost 40% of all pain episodes in children with cancer attributed to?
    a. Separation from parents
    b. Procedures
    c. Separation from peers
    d. Hospitalization

52. What is the most common clinical syndrome of neuropathic pain?

53. Abdominal pain after allogeneic bone marrow transplantation may be associated with what acute disease?
    a. Graft-versus-host
    b. Typhlitis
    c. Phantom limb pain
    d. Medullary bone pain

Pain and Sedation in End-of-Life Care

54. Why would a continuing high-dose infusion of opioids along with sedation be prescribed in end-of-life care?

APPLYING CRITICAL THINKING TO THE NURSING PRACTICE

A. Valery, age 7, comes into the acute care center of the local children's hospital. She has been hurt in an automobile accident. On assessment, the nurse notices she has multiple bruises on her head, shoulder, and right knee. X-ray studies reveal she has dislocated her right knee and right shoulder. She is screaming in pain. Her mother and father were also in the vehicle but uninjured. Just before the accident, Valery had taken off her seatbelt to grab a piece of paper off the floor of the car. She has rated her pain at 9 on a scale from 0 to 10, with 10 being the most extreme pain and 0 being the least amount of pain. She has an elevated heart rate of 100 beats/min, blood pressure of 150/99 mm Hg, and respirations of 18 breaths/min. She is also talking very fast and has a stiff body posture. You are a nursing student assigned to assist the nurse in the care for Valery during the first morning shift after her accident. Answer the following questions pertaining to the nursing care for Valery.
    1. What behavioral symptoms would the nurse notice when using the FLACC to further assess Valery's pain? What other tool, involving her parents, could the nurse use as a secondary resource for evaluating Valery's pain?

    2. Describe at least five physiologic parameters that could give the nurse additional information on the severity of her pain.

3. The physician prescribed a combination of nonsteroidal antiinflammatory drugs (NSAIDs) and opioids for optimum pain relief. Why is this a preferred treatment of severe pain?

4. Based on your assessment data, what adjuvant therapy can you anticipate the physician will prescribe for these symptoms?

B. You are a nursing student assigned to care for a 4-year-old boy, Simon. When you arrive to care for him, he is just getting back from surgery. You find out in the report that he had an emergency appendectomy. His mother and father are in the room with him. On assessment, you note he appears frightened and is clenching his jaw. His eyebrows are furrowed, and his forehead is wrinkled. He is wiggling his toes, and his respirations seem slightly labored. With movement, his eyes get more pronounced and he cries.
1. What is the first thing you need to assess in Simon? How would you assess this?

2. What kind of complication can occur after any type of abdominal surgery that could affect his airway and breathing?

3. How can acute pain further complicate his recovery process?

4. Based on the assessment data, what would the priority nursing diagnosis be?

C. You are a nursing student caring for a 7-year-old boy, Sajin, who has come to the clinic to receive his annual flu vaccine. What expected response to receiving an injection should you be prepared to see in a child his age?

D. Damon is an 11-year-old boy who just received a lumbar puncture for administration of chemotherapy. Damon is now complaining of a painful headache. What is an appropriate nursing intervention for alleviating headache after lumbar puncture?

6 | Infectious Disease

REVIEW OF ESSENTIAL CONCEPTS

1. Which of the following is a preventable condition if caregivers practice meticulous cleaning and disposal techniques?
   a. Standard precautions
   b. Hospital-acquired infections (HAIs)
   c. Pertussis
   d. Measles

2. The nurse caring for infants in the neonatal intensive care unit recognizes that the single most important practice to reduce the transmission of infectious diseases is
   a. implementing standard precautions.
   b. wearing disposable gloves.
   c. hand hygiene.
   d. implementing airborne precautions.

3. Match the following statements to the correct description

   a. _____ Airborne precautions

   b. _____ Droplet precautions

   c. _____ Direct contact precautions

   d. _____ Indirect contact precautions

   1. Involves contact of the conjunctivae or mucous membranes of the nose or mouth of a susceptible person
   2. Involves contact of a susceptible host with a contaminated intermediate object in the patient's environment
   3. Involves skin-to-skin contact and physical transfer of microorganisms to a susceptible host from an infected or colonized person
   4. Involves dissemination of droplet nuclei or dust particles containing the infectious agent

4. Which of the following is the most potent source of harmful microorganisms and nosocomial infections?
   a. Medication station
   b. Lunch room
   c. Blood pressure machines
   d. Stethoscopes

5. What is the recommended age for beginning primary immunizations of infants?
   a. At birth
   b. By 6 months of age
   c. By 2 months of age
   d. Anytime within the infant's first year

6. Which of the following conditions can hepatitis B virus infections cause?
   a. Heart disease
   b. Urinary cancer
   c. Cirrhosis or liver cancer
   d. Diabetes

7. The nurse is caring for a child diagnosed with hepatitis A. The nurse recognizes that hepatitis A is spread
   a. via air droplets.
   b. via fecal-oral route.
   c. via immunizations.
   d. via surgery.

8. What is the cutaneous manifestations of diphtheria?
   a. Muscle atrophy
   b. Abdominal distention
   c. Headache and seizures
   d. Skin lesions

9. At what age should the tetanus vaccine be given?
   a. 11 to 12 years old
   b. 8 to 10 years old
   c. 12 to 14 years old
   d. 10 to 12 years old

10. How many doses of inactivated poliovirus vaccine should all children receive?
    a. One
    b. Two
    c. Three
    d. Four

11. The administration of _____ has been effective in decreasing the morbidity and mortality associated with measles in developing countries.
    a. vitamin A
    b. vitamin B
    c. vitamin D
    d. vitamin K

12. Which vaccine protects against a number of serious infections including bacterial meningitis, epiglottitis, and sepsis?
    a. Rubella
    b. Tetanus
    c. *Haemophilus influenzae* type b
    d. Varicella

13. The nurse recognizes that the use of meningococcal and diphtheria proteins in combination vaccines does not mean the child has received adequate immunization for meningococcal or diphtheria illnesses. What must the child be given to protect against these diseases?
    a. Two combination vaccines
    b. The appropriate vaccine for that specific disease
    c. Vaccines spaced 3 months apart
    d. Vaccines spaced 6 months apart

14. The nurse is preparing to give a 12-month-old boy his first dose of varicella. How is this medication administered?
    a. Via oral route
    b. Via intranasal route
    c. Via subcutaneous route
    d. Via intramuscular route

15. Which childhood vaccine provides protection against otitis media, sinusitis, and pneumonia?
    a. Pneumococcal vaccine
    b. MMR vaccine
    c. Tetanus vaccine
    d. Rubella vaccine

16. Which of the following vaccines is recommended annually for children 6 months to 18 years of age?
    a. MMR vaccine
    b. Varicella
    c. Pneumococcal vaccine
    d. Influenza vaccine

17. _____ is the leading cause of bacterial meningitis in the United States.
    a. *Listeria monocytogenes*
    b. *Haemophilus influenzae*
    c. *Neisseria meningitidis*
    d. *Cryptococcus neoformans*

18. One of the leading causes of severe diarrhea in infants and young children is
    a. pneumonia.
    b. pneumococcal disease.
    c. rotovirus.
    d. measles.

19. The nurse administers routine vaccines to a child. Within minutes, the child develops tachycardia, hypertension, irritability, and nausea. What type of reaction is the child having?
    a. A mild reaction
    b. A moderate reaction
    c. An adverse reaction
    d. A normal response

20. Which vaccine is associated with a low-grade fever and mild local reaction at the site of injection?
    a. Rotavirus vaccine
    b. Hib vaccine
    c. Pneumococcal vaccine
    d. MMR

21. An infant comes to the clinic to receive her scheduled immunizations. Upon assessment, the nurse notes that the infant has a low-grade fever, congestion, and nasal drainage. Which of the following is the most appropriate intervention?
    a. Withhold the vaccines until the infant is healthy.
    b. Administer the vaccines to ensure that the infant stays on schedule.
    c. Treat the symptoms first, then administer the scheduled vaccines.
    d. If the child has had the symptoms for less than 24 hours, administer the vaccines.

22. Which of the following are contraindications to receiving a live virus vaccine?
    a. A child who received a recent blood transfusion
    b. A severely immunocompromised child
    c. A child with severe febrile illness
    d. All of the above

Communicable Diseases

23. The most common preventative measure for disease and the control of its spread to others is
    a. primary prevention.
    b. secondary prevention.
    d. tertiary prevention.
    e. education.

24. Children who have had varicella are at risk for developing what disease?
    a. Viremia
    b. Herpes zoster
    c. Bacterial infection
    d. Measles

25. What medication is used to treat varicella infections in susceptible immunocompromised persons?
    a. Relenza (zanamivir)
    b. Tamiflu (oseltamivir phosphate)
    c. Flumadine (rimantadine)
    d. Acyclovir (Zovirax)

26. What are early clinical manifestations of pertussis in infants?
    a. Gagging, coughing, emesis, and apnea
    b. Hypertension, emesis, and nausea
    c. Coughing, fever, and apnea
    d. Gagging, hypertension, and apnea

27. Prevention of complications from diseases such as diphtheria, pertussis, and scarlet fever requires compliance with

    _____ therapy.
    a. respiratory
    b. antibiotic
    c. chest physio
    d. antiviral

28. Which of the following is the most effective nursing intervention for the child who presents with a rash and itching?
    a. Cool baths and calming lotions
    b. Fresh sheets and hot compresses
    c. Warm baths and distraction methods
    d. Distraction and play therapy

29. An infant presents with recurrent conjunctivitis. The nurse recognizes that this may be a sign of
    a. a chemical injury.
    b. a nasolacrimal (tear) duct obstruction.
    c. a foreign body.
    d. pneumonia.

30. What is the most appropriate way to remove accumulated secretions from the eye?
    a. Wiping from the outer canthus downward and outward, away from the opposite eye
    b. Wiping from the inner canthus downward and outward, toward the opposite eye
    c. Wiping from the inner canthus downward and outward, away from the opposite eye
    d. Wiping from the outer canthus downward and outward, toward the opposite eye

31. _____ is the inflammation of the oral mucosa, which may include the buccal and labial mucosa, tongue, gingiva, palate, and floor of the mouth.
    a. Herpes zoster
    b. Herpes simplex
    c. Stomatitis
    d. Gingivitis

32. A child presents with vesicles on the buccal mucosa and refuses to take the bottle. The nurse recognizes that this is a common symptom of children who present with
    a. hand-foot-mouth disease.
    b. varicella.
    c. impetigo.
    d. tinea capitis.

33. _____ constitute the most frequent infections in the world.

34. What are the two most common parasitic infections among children in the United States?
    a. Giardiasis and bacterial infections
    b. Giardiasis and pinworms
    c. Pinworms and bacterial infections
    d. Giardiasis and viral infections

35. One of the most common intestinal parasitic pathogens in the United States acquired from a contaminated water source is
    a. *Giardia intestinalis.*
    b. enterobiasis.
    c. *Rotavirus.*
    d. *Staphylococcus aureus.*

36. A nurse caring for a child with suspected giardiasis encourages the child to swallow a gelatin capsule in order to
    a. perform a biopsy.
    b. perform a string test.
    c. direct aspiration.
    d. none of the above.

37. What is the most important nursing consideration in the care of the child with giardiasis?
    a. Education of the parents
    b. Attention to the child's environment
    c. Prevention of giardiasis
    d. Prevention of giardiasis and education of parents

38. _____ is the most common helminthic infection in the United States.

39. A child who goes to day care has recently been complaining of intense rectal itching. What is a common cause of intense rectal itching in children?

40. How are pinworms diagnosed?

41. When should the nurse direct the parents to collect pinworm specimens?
    a. After the child has a bowel movement
    b. After a bath
    c. When the child goes to sleep
    d. As the child awakens

Bacterial Infections
42. What is the major nursing function related to bacterial skin infections?
    a. To treat the infection
    b. To minimize pain
    c. To prevent the spread of infection
    d. To treat complications

Viral Infections
43. Infections caused by a group of closely related filamentous fungi that invade primarily the stratum corneum, hair, and nails is referred to as
    a. pediculosis capitis.
    b. mycotic.
    c. enterobiasis.
    d. dermatophytoses.

44. _____ is an endemic infestation caused by mites.

45. _____ is a common parasite in school-age children.

46. A child presents with bedbugs. What are some common clinical manifestations of this condition?
    a. Erythematous papule, rash, vesicles, and urticaria
    b. Rash, nausea, irritation, redness
    c. Nausea, rash, vesicles, urticaria
    d. Bullae, nausea, rash, and urticaria

APPLYING CRITICAL THINKING TO THE NURSING PRACTICE

A. A 7-year-old boy presents to the clinic with a history of irritability, headaches, insomnia, anorexia, generalized lymphadenopathy, and sore throat. The child lives in a wooded area and often plays outside with his brothers. Answer the following questions regarding this assessment.
    1. What possible condition could the boy have based on the assessment data?

    2. How is this disease diagnosed?

    3. How is this disease treated?

    4. What should be the major emphasis of nursing care in this case?

B. A child presents with a painless, nonpruritic erythematous papule at the site of inoculation, followed by regional lymphadenitis. The child is diagnosed with cat scratch disease. Answer the following questions regarding this assessment.
    1. What lymph nodes does the nurse expect to be most commonly involved with this disease?

    2. What are some potential serious complications of this disease?

    3. What three criteria is the diagnosis based on?

7 Health Promotion of the Newborn and Family

Chapter 7 introduces the factors the nurse must consider when caring for the newborn and family during delivery and the neonatal period. After completing this chapter, the student will understand the fundamentals for providing nursing care for the neonate and family. This knowledge will enable the student to assess and formulate nursing goals and interventions that facilitate normal physiologic and psychologic adjustment and development in the newborn and family.

REVIEW OF ESSENTIAL CONCEPTS

Adjustment to Extrauterine Life

1. Indicate whether each of the following statements is true or false.
   a. **T F** The most profound physiologic change required of the neonate is the transition from fetal or placental circulation to independent respiration.
   b. **T F** The most critical and immediate physiologic change required of the newborn is the onset of thermoregulation.
   c. **T F** The stimuli that help initiate the first respiration are primarily chemical and thermal.
   d. **T F** A change in the cardiovascular system that occurs after birth involves an increase in pressure in the right atrium of the heart.

2. Which of the following is the most important factor in controlling the closure of the ductus arteriosus?
   a. Increased oxygen concentration of the blood
   b. Deposition of fibrin and cells
   c. Rise of endogenous prostaglandin
   d. Presence of metabolic acidosis

3. Which of the following factors predispose the neonate to heat loss?
   a. Small surface area, thin layer of subcutaneous fat, inability to shiver
   b. Large surface area, thick layer of subcutaneous fat, inability to shiver
   c. Large surface area, thin layer of subcutaneous fat, inability to shiver
   d. Small surface area, thick layer of subcutaneous fat, inability to shiver

4. Why is it essential that newly born infants be quickly dried and either provided with warm, dry blankets or placed skin-to-skin with the mother after delivery?

5. The infant's rate of metabolism is _____ as great as that of the adult, relative to body weight.
   a. one time
   b. two times
   c. three times
   d. four times

6. What enzyme is contained in human milk?
   a. Lipase
   b. Lactoferrin
   c. Lysozyme
   d. Caritine

7. Which of the following limits a newborn's gastrointestinal system?
   a. The large volume of the colon
   b. A decreased number of secretory glands
   c. An increased gastric capacity
   d. A lower esophageal sphincter pressure

8. All structural components are present in the renal system of a newborn, but there is a functional deficiency in the

   kidney's ability to _____ and to cope with conditions of fluid and electrolyte stress, such as dehydration or a concentrated solute load.
   a. detoxify medications
   b. concentrate urine
   c. dilute urine
   d. maintain pH

9. Plugging of the sebaceous glands causes _____.

10. What are the infant's three lines of defense against infection?
   a.

   b.

   c.

11. In the newborn, the pituitary gland's posterior lobe produces limited quantities of antidiuretic hormone, or vasopressin, which inhibits diuresis. This renders the young infant highly susceptible to
   a. muscle loss.
   b. urinary retention.
   c. dehydration.
   d. urinary tract infections.

12. Indicate whether each of the following statements is true or false.
   a. **T   F**   At birth, the eye is structurally complete.
   b. **T   F**   After the amniotic fluid has drained from the ears, the infant probably has auditory acuity similar to that of an adult.
   c. **T   F**   Infants are able to differentiate the breast milk of their mother from the breast milk of other women by smell.
   d. **T   F**   During early childhood, the taste buds are not yet developed, preventing the newborn from distinguishing between tastes.
   e. **T   F**   The face (especially the mouth), hands, and soles of the feet seem to be most sensitive to touch in infancy.

Nursing Care of the Newborn and Family
13. The Apgar score is comprised of the following five elements:
   a.

   b.

   c.

d.

e.

14. What is the maximum score an infant can receive on the Apgar?
    a. 8
    b. 9
    c. 10
    d. 11

15. Which two factors of infants at birth are used to predict morbidity and mortality risks?
    a.

    b.

16. Indicate whether each of the following statements is true or false.
    a. **T** **F** The normal head circumference of the neonate is 48 to 53 cm (19 to 21 inches).
    b. **T** **F** Head circumference is usually about 2 to 3 cm (about 1 inch) greater than chest circumference.
    c. **T** **F** Normally the neonate loses about 20% of birth weight by 3 or 4 days of age.
    d. **T** **F** Tympanic thermometers have been found to be more accurate than temporal artery thermometers.
    e. **T** **F** The normal pulse rate of the neonate is 120 to 140 beats/min.
    f. **T** **F** Respirations and pulse rate are counted for a full 60 seconds to detect irregularities in rate or rhythm.

17. The nurse in labor and delivery is caring for an infant who was just born. Which of the following phases of the assessment should the nurse initially provide to the newly delivered infant?
    a. The initial assessment, which includes the Apgar scoring system
    b. Transitional assessment during the periods of reactivity
    c. Assessment of gestational age
    d. Systematic physical examination

18. Of the following responses, which reflex is present in a healthy neonate?
    a. Landau
    b. Moro
    c. Parachute
    d. Neck-righting

19. Both the anterior and posterior fontanels should feel _____ and well demarcated against the bony edges of the skull.
    a. sunken and soft
    b. flat and soft
    c. sunken and firm
    d. flat and firm

20. _____ is a normal finding that results from the newborn's lack of binocularity of the eyes.

21. Describe how the nurse would elicit the rooting reflex in an infant.

22. What would the plan of action be if, on auscultation of the newborn a few hours after birth, the nurse hears lung sounds with wheezes or medium or coarse crackles along with stridor?

23. Bowel sounds should be heard within the first _____ minutes after birth.
    a. 5 to 10
    b. 10
    c. 15 to 20
    d. 30 to 45

24. _____ is a manifestation of the abrupt decrease of maternal hormones within the mother and usually disappears by 2 to 4 weeks.

25. In small newborn males, particularly preterm infants, the _____ may be palpable within the inguinal canal.
    a. undescended testes
    b. hernia
    c. spermatic cord
    d. hydrocele

26. A protruding sac anywhere along the spine, but most commonly in the sacral area, indicates some type of
    a. hydrocele.
    b. hernia.
    c. spina bifida.
    d. meningitis.

27. What could asymmetry of muscle tone indicate?

Transitional Assessment: Periods of Reactivity

28. What is the first period of reactivity?
    a. 4 to 6 hours after birth
    b. 6 to 8 hours after birth
    c. 2 to 3 hours after birth
    d. 5 to 7 hours after birth

29. Which of the following occurs during the second period of reactivity?
    a. An alert and active infant, increased heart and respiratory rate, active gag reflex
    b. Increased gastric and respiratory secretions, and decreased respiratory rate
    c. Passage of meconium, decreased gastric and respiratory secretions
    d. An alert and active infant, passage of meconium, and decreased respiratory rate

30. What is the Brazelton Neonatal Behavioral Assessment Scale (BNBAS)?

31. A new mom comes into the clinic. Upon history she states that her infant sleeps 10 hours in a 24-hour time period. Which of the following interventions does the nurse need to implement in this case?
    a. Nothing. The intake history meets current sleep recommendations.
    b. Educate the mother that infants need 14 to hours of sleep in a 24-hour time period.
    c. Educate the mother that infants need 16 to 18 hours of sleep in a 24-hour time period.
    d. Educate the mother that infants need 12 to 15 hours of sleep in a 24-hour time period.

Assessment of Attachment Behaviors

32. Name four attachment behaviors.
    a.

    b.

    c.

    d.

Physical Assessment

33. What is the primary objective immediately after delivery?
    a. Drying off the infant and establishing a warm environment
    b. Assessing neurologic function
    c. Assessing circulation
    d. Establishing a patent airway

34. Identify the five cardinal signs of respiratory distress in the newborn.
    a.

    b.

    c.

    d.

    e.

35. Identify four major causes of heat loss at birth.
    a.

    b.

c.

d.

Protection from Infection and Injury

36. The most important practice for preventing cross-infection is thorough _____.

37. The nurse needs to discuss safety issues with the mother the first time the infant is brought to her. The National

Center for Missing and Exploited Children (NCMEC) has reported that _____ of infant abductions occur in the mother's room.
    a. 12%
    b. 32%
    c. 58%
    d. 78%

38. Describe the typical profile of an infant abductor.

39. A nurse is caring for an infant who received ophthalmic prophylaxis 18 hours ago. What clinical features can indicate that the newborn has chemical conjunctivitis?
    a. Redness and irritation
    b. Purulent eye discharge with no evidence of lid edema
    c. Nonpurulent eye discharge and redness
    d. Nonpurulent eye discharge and mild lid edema

40. Why is vitamin K administered to the newborn?

41. What is the nurse's responsibility regarding newborn screening for disease?

42. What forms the skin's "acid mantle"?

43. The average umbilical cord separation time is _____ to _____ days.

44. Indicate whether each of the following statements is true or false.
    a. **T F** When undergoing circumcision, infants need no anesthesia because they feel no pain.
    b. **T F** Normally, on the second day after circumcision, a yellowish white exudate forms as part of the granulation process.

Provision of Optimum Nutrition

45. Why is breast milk more easily digestible to the newborn?

46. What five conditions has human milk been proven, through research, to protect the newborn from?
    a.

    b.

    c.

    d.

    e.

47. What five factors have been implicated in the decline of breastfeeding after discharge from the hospital?
    a.

    b.

    c.

    d.

    e.

48. What has the American Academy of Pediatrics stated as its position on breastfeeding?

49. Successful breastfeeding depends on which three factors?

    a.

    b.

    c.

50. List the three main criteria that have been proposed as essential in promoting positive breastfeeding.

    a.

    b.

    c.

51. What can nurses teach new mothers who choose to bottle feed their infant to help ensure the emotional component of feeding?

52. The nurse enters the room to find the infant in the bassinet with a bottle propped up while the mother is on the phone with her husband. What nursing intervention is most important for the nurse to provide in this situation?

    a. Educate the mother on the importance of breastfeeding.

    b. Teach the mother the proper ways of propping a bottle.

    c. Educate the mother on the dangers of bottle propping.

    d. Teach the mother that bottle propping is okay as long as she is holding the infant.

53. Identify the four categories of commercially prepared infant formulas.

    a.

    b.

    c.

    d.

54. The infant is making sucking movements and rooting. The nurse recognizes this to be the _____ of the five behavioral stages that occur during successful feeding.

    a. prefeeding

    b. approach

    c. attachment

    d. consummatory

55. Describe two ways nurses can positively influence the attachment of parent and child.

a.

b.

56. The nurse is caring for a mother on day 2 postdelivery of a healthy boy. Upon reading the mother's medical record, the nurse noted a history of depression. Which of the following observations could indicate possible depression in the mother of a newly delivered infant?

a. The mother talks and laughs about how the boy looks like her husband.
b. The mother is on her phone talking to her mother the majority of the time.
c. When the nurse hands the mother her baby, the mother has minimal eye contact with the baby.
d. The mother changes the baby's diaper and asks about care of the baby's umbilical cord.

57. Identify at least four ways a nurse can encourage the father's engrossment.

a.

b.

c.

d.

58. What is the most important principle for the nurse to assist parents of twins in the bonding process?

Preparation for Discharge and Home Care

59. When does discharge teaching for the new family begin?

60. Why are discharge planning and care at home of increasing importance?

61. Infants who weigh less than 9.07 kg (20 pounds) or who are younger than _____ should always be placed in a rear-facing child safety seat in the car's back seat.

A. You are a new nursing student who has performed the initial assessment on a newborn. Answer the following questions regarding that assessment.
   1. The infant received a score of irregular, slow, weak cry under respiratory effort and a 1 under the Apgar's heart rate category. This indicates that the neonate's heart rate was _____.

   2. Name at least one factor that could affect a newborn's Apgar score.

   3. On assessment, you noted that the infant appeared to be alert, cried vigorously, sucked his fist, and seemed interested in his surroundings. How would you describe the infant's state of activity?

   4. Which of the following is an appropriate nursing intervention in the first stage of reactivity?
      a. Giving the initial bath
      b. Administering eyedrops before the child has contact with the parents
      c. Encouraging the mother to breastfeed
      d. Minimizing contact with the parents until the child's temperature has stabilized

B. The following questions relate to determining a neonate's gestational age.
   1. Why is it important to know the neonate's gestational age?

   2. What six neuromuscular signs are assessed to determine gestational age?
      a.

      b.

      c.

      d.

      e.

      f.

   3. After plotting the infant's height, weight, and head circumference on standardized graphs, you determine that the infant is normal for gestational age because _____.

C. The following questions relate to the stooling patterns of newborns.

    1. The first stool is called _____. Describe the characteristics of this stool.

    2. The transitional stool is characterized by what features?

    3. Differentiate between breastfed and bottle-fed infant stools.

D. The following questions relate to a newborn's physical assessment.
    1. What should you suspect if the head circumference is significantly smaller than the crown-rump length?

    2. You note an absence of arm movement on range of motion of the left arm. What could be the cause for this finding?

E. Baby boy Keating is a 1-day-old infant who is rooming in with his mother. Baby Keating is a full-term healthy infant who received a normal newborn examination. Baby boy Keating is the first child to his mother.
    1. Formulate at least three nursing diagnoses for Baby Keating during the newborn period.
      a.

      b.

      c.

    2. List at least four nursing interventions that should be used to maintain a patent airway in Baby Keating.
      a.

      b.

      c.

      d.

3. What criteria could be used to evaluate nursing interventions aimed at maintaining a patent airway in the transition period?

4. What areas should be included in the discharge planning of Baby Keating and his parents?

8 Health Problems of Newborns

Chapter 8 addresses common health problems in the newborn, including birth injuries and high-risk neonatal care. This chapter outlines nursing care related to prematurity, postmaturity, and physiologic factors. Nursing care of newborns related to infectious processes and maternal conditions is also presented. After completing this chapter, the student will be able to formulate nursing goals and interventions to provide for the normal development of the newborn and to assist the family in coping with the stress of a neonatal health problem.

REVIEW OF ESSENTIAL CONCEPTS

Birth Injuries

1. Which of the following increases the risk of a subgaleal brain hemorrhage?
   a. C-section section delivery
   b. Breech delivery
   c. Vacuum extraction delivery
   d. Complicated delivery

2. What is an early sign of a subgaleal brain hemorrhage?
   a. A boggy fluctuant mass over the scalp that crosses the suture line
   b. Pallor and fussiness in the baby
   c. Tachycardia and decreasing head circumference
   d. Bradycardia and increasing head circumference

3. Any newborn who is large for its gestational age or weighs more than 3855 g (8.5 pounds) and is delivered vaginally

   should be evaluated for a(n) _____.

4. A neonate exhibits loss of movement on one side of the face and an absence of wrinkling of the forehead. What does this assessment suggest?

Common Problems in the Newborn

5. Match the following statements with the correct response.

   a. _____ Erythema toxicum neonatorum

   b. _____ Neonatal herpes

   c. _____ Candidiasis

   1. This yeastlike fungus (it produces yeast cells and spores) can be acquired from a maternal vaginal infection during delivery; by person-to-person transmission (especially poor hand-washing technique); or from contaminated hands, bottles, nipples, or other articles.
   2. Lesions are firm, 1- to 3-mm, pale yellow or white papules or pustules on an erythematous base; they resemble flea bites.
   3. This manifests in one of three ways: with skin, eye, and mouth involvement; as a localized central nervous system disease; or as a disseminated disease involving multiple organs. In skin and eye disease, a rash appears as vesicles or pustules on an erythematous base.

6. Match each type of birthmark with its definition.

a. _____ Capillary hemangioma

b. _____ Port-wine stains

c. _____ Café au lait spots

d. _____ Cavernous venous hemangioma

1. Involves deep vessels in the dermis, is a bluish-red color, and has poorly defined margins
2. Multiple light brown discolorations, often associated with autosomal dominant hereditary disorders
3. Pink, red, or purple stains of the skin that thicken, darken, and enlarge as the child grows
4. Benign cutaneous tumor that involves only capillaries

Nursing Care of the High-Risk Newborn and Family

7. A(n) _____ can be defined as a newborn, regardless of gestational age or birth weight, who has a greater-than-average chance of morbidity or mortality because of conditions or circumstances superimposed on the normal course of events associated with birth and the adjustment to extrauterine existence.

8. How are high-risk newborns classified?

9. Although most high-risk newborns are monitored by equipment with an alarm system that indicates when the vital signs are above or below preset limits, it is essential to check the _____ and compare it with the monitor reading.

10. Which of the following ways can a nurse obtain an accurate output in high-risk newborns?
    a. By collecting urine in a plastic urine collection bag specifically made for premature infants
    b. By inserting a clean intermittent catheter
    c. By suprapubic aspiration
    d. By recording the intakes and outputs on the medical record

11. What is the primary objective in the care of high-risk infants?
    a. Cardiovascular support
    b. Thermoregulation
    c. To establish and maintain respiration
    d. To provide family-centered care

12. Prevention of heat loss in the distressed infant is absolutely essential for survival. Maintaining a(n) _____ is a challenging aspect of neonatal intensive nursing care.

13. Identify the three consequences of cold stress.
    a.

    b.

    c.

14. Identify two ways nurses monitor fluid status in high-risk newborns.

    a.

    b.

15. A nurse caring for an infant notices that the infant has a weight gain of 32 g in 24 hours, periorbital edema, tachypnea, and crackles on lung auscultation. What do these findings suggest?
    a. Dehydration
    b. Adequate hydration
    c. Overhydration
    d. Edema

16. Why are infants highly prone to aspiration and its attendant dangers?
    a. Because breast milk can be difficult for the infant to digest
    b. Because formula can be difficult for the infant to digest
    c. Because initial sucking is not accompanied by swallowing
    d. Because the swallowing mechanism exists before initial sucking

17. What factor has been associated with enteral feedings in acutely ill or distressed infants?
    a. Hypoxia
    b. Septicemia
    c. Necrotizing enterocolitis
    d. Dehydration

18. Because of the antiinfective and growth-promoting properties of human milk, as well as its superior nutrition,

    _____ is used in many neonatal intensive care units (NICUs) for preterm or sick infants when the mother's milk is not available.

19. The amount and method of feeding the preterm infant are determined by the infant's _____

    and _____ of previous feeding.

20. Which of the following does the nurse understand that a developmental approach to feeding considers?
    a. The individual infant's response to feeding
    b. The individual infant's readiness for feeding
    c. The individual infant's pattern of feeding
    d. The individual infant's style of feeding

21. Which of the following suggests poor feeding behaviors such as apnea, bradycardia, cyanosis, pallor, and decreased oxygen saturation in any infant who has previously fed well?
    a. An underlying illness
    b. Cancer
    c. Aspiration
    d. A cardiovascular defect

22. What are the five signs that indicate readiness for oral feedings in high-risk neonates?
    a.

    b.

    c.

d.

e.

23. Early in hospitalization, the _____ position is best for most preterm infants and results in improved oxygenation, better-tolerated feedings, and more organized sleep-rest patterns.

24. Recommendations for protecting the integrity of premature skin include using minimal adhesive tape, backing the tape with cotton, and which of the following?
    a. Using an alcohol wipe to remove adhesive and pectin barrier
    b. Removing adhesive and pectin barrier simultaneously
    c. Delaying adhesive and pectin barrier removal until adherence is reduced
    d. Removing adhesive and pectin barrier swiftly in one motion to avoid contamination

25. What is a common preservative in bacteriostatic water and saline that has been shown to be toxic to newborns? Products containing this preservative should not be used to flush IV catheters, to dilute or reconstitute medications, or to use as an anesthetic when starting IVs.
    a. Bacteriostatic solutions
    b. Hyperosmolar products
    c. Preservatives
    d. Benzyl alcohol

26. Which of the following are major benefits of skin-to-skin contact for neonates?
    a. Reduced risk of mortality, fewer nosocomial infections, increased length of hospital stay
    b. Maintenance of neonatal thermal stability and oxygen saturation, increased feeding vigor, and reduced growth
    c. Reduced risk of mortality, increase risk of nosocomial infections, decreased length of hospital stay
    d. Maintenance of neonatal thermal stability and oxygen saturation, increased feeding vigor, and increased growth

27. A nurse is performing an initial assessment on a newborn. The nurse notes decreased Pao_2, increased Pco_2, pounding peripheral pulses, and a systolic murmur. What do these clinical manifestations suggest?
    a. Vitamin K deficiency
    b. Hypoxic-ischemic brain injury
    c. Patent ductus arteriosus
    d. Intracranial hemorrhage

28. List two ways personnel can reduce noise in the NICU.
    a.

    b.

29. List two ways personnel can establish a night-day sleep pattern for infants in the NICU.
    a.

    b.

Chapter **8** **Health Problems of Newborns**

30. To alleviate distress in NICU infants, _____ may be used before invasive procedures, such as heel stick.
   a. swaddling the infant
   b. turning on soft music
   c. giving the infant a pacifier
   d. reducing noise levels in the unit

31. The nurse is caring for an infant who was just admitted to the NICU. Before the parents first visit to the neonatal unit, what should the nurse do to prepare the parents?
   a. Have the parents watch a video of what takes place in the NICU.
   b. Discuss the infant's appearance and the equipment attached to the child and give some indication of the unit's general atmosphere.
   c. Assure the parents that their infant will only be in the NICU for 24 to 48 hours for stabilization.
   d. Register the parents for infant care classes and cardiopulmonary resuscitation (CPR).

32. _____ is the first act of communication between parents and child.
   a. Seeing
   b. Hearing
   c. Touching
   d. Longing

33. In neonatal loss, it is important for the nurse to help parents understand that the death is a reality by encouraging the family to _____ their infant before death and, if possible, to _____ at the time of death so that their infant can die in their arms if they choose.
   a. hold, be present
   b. touch, take pictures
   c. see, be present
   d. see, take pictures

High Risk Related to Dysmaturity

34. Match each characteristic with its corresponding type of maturity.

   a. _____ Minimal subcutaneous fat deposits

   b. _____ Presence of subcutaneous fat

   c. _____ Cracked and parchmentlike skin

   1. Preterm
   2. Postmature
   3. Term

High Risk Related to Physiologic Factors

35. An infant presents to the nursery with yellow skin and yellow in the sclera of both eyes. Labs reveal an excessive level of accumulated bilirubin in the blood. What do these clinical manifestations suggest?
   a. Cytomegalovirus
   b. Hepatosplenomegaly
   c. Hyperbilirubinemia
   d. Hypobilirubinemia

36. What is the most common cause of hyperbilirubinemia in newborns?
   a. Breastfeeding
   b. Mother with diabetes
   c. Enzyme deficiency
   d. Physiologic jaundice

37. What is the most common treatment for hyperbilirubinemia?
   a. Phototherapy
   b. Hydration
   c. Cessation of breastfeeding
   d. Scheduled feedings

38. What is often the cause of hyperbilirubinemia in the first 24 hours of life?
    a. Hypothyroidism
    b. Rh incompatibilities
    c. Blood incompatibilities
    d. Hemolytic disease of the newborn

39. The most common blood group incompatibility in the neonate is between a mother with blood

    type _____ and an infant with type _____ or

    _____ blood.

40. _____, in which the infant's blood is removed in small amounts (usually 5 to 10 ml at a time) and replaced with compatible blood (such as Rh-negative blood), is a standard mode of therapy for treatment of severe hyperbilirubinemia and is the treatment of choice for hyperbilirubinemia and hydrops caused by Rh incompatibility.

41. Which of the following is a factor in the pathophysiology of respiratory distress syndrome?
    a. Decreased pulmonary vascular resistance
    b. Increase in pulmonary blood flow
    c. Deficient production of surfactant
    d. Respiratory alkalosis

42. What are the three goals of oxygen therapy?
    a.

    b.

    c.

43. Which of the following are the most advantageous positions for maintaining an infant's open airway?
    a. On the side with the head supported in alignment by a small folded blanket, or prone positioned to keep the neck slightly extended
    b. On the side with the head supported in alignment by a small folded blanket, or, when on the back, positioned to keep the neck slightly extended
    c. Prone with the head supported in alignment by a small folded blanket, or, when on the back, positioned to keep the neck slightly extended
    d. Supine with the head supported in alignment by a small folded blanket, or, when on the back, positioned to keep the neck slightly extended

44. The most serious cardiovascular disorders of the newborn are _____ defects.
    a. anemia
    b. respiratory distress
    c. congenital heart
    d. seizures

45. Seizures in the neonatal period are usually the clinical manifestation of a(n)
    a. infection.
    b. severe allergy.
    c. neurologic injury.
    d. serious underlying disease.

46. What is the most prominent feature of neurologic dysfunction in the neonatal period?

47. _____ is acquired in the perinatal period; infection can occur from direct contact with organisms from the maternal gastrointestinal and genitourinary tracts.
    a. Rh factor
    b. Cytomegalovirus
    c. Early-onset sepsis
    d. Late-onset sepsis

48. What is the most common infecting organism in term infants?
    a. *Escherichia coli*
    b. Group B streptococcus
    c. *Treponema pallidum*
    d. Toxoplasmosis

49. Which of the following are central nervous system signs of neonatal sepsis?
    a. Dyspnea
    b. Full fontanel
    c. Mottling
    d. Hypothermia

50. Define *necrotizing enterocolitis* (NEC).

51. Identify three factors that play a significant role in the development of NEC.
    a.

    b.

    c.

52. Identify at least four specific signs of NEC.
    a.

    b.

    c.

    d.

High Risk Related to Maternal Conditions

53. What is the single most important factor influencing the fetal well-being when the mother is diabetic?

54. Elevated levels of hemoglobin A1c during the _____ trimester appear to be associated with a higher incidence of congenital malformations.
   a. second
   b. first
   c. third
   d. all of the above

55. Which of the following is a characteristic clinical manifestation of an infant whose mother's diabetes is not under complete control?
   a. Hyperglycemia
   b. Loss of subcutaneous fat
   c. Absence of vernix caseosa
   d. Large for gestational age

56. An infant presents with the following clinical manifestations: sucking avidly on fists, displaying an exaggerated rooting reflex, and uncoordinated and ineffectual sucking and swallowing reflexes. What do these clinical manifestations suggest?
   a. Drug-narcotic exposure
   b. Adverse reaction to medications
   c. Digestion or intestinal problems
   d. Normal signs of hunger

57. Which of the following is the most accurate for determining whether an infant was exposed to drugs in utero?
   a. Urine toxicology
   b. Blood sampling
   c. Meconium sampling
   d. Saliva testing

58. What are common findings of infants exposed to cocaine in utero?
   a. Preterm birth, a larger head circumference, increased birth length, and decreased weight
   b. Preterm birth, a smaller head circumference, decreased birth length, and decreased weight
   c. Preterm birth, a smaller head circumference, increased birth length, and decreased weight
   d. Preterm birth, a smaller head circumference, decreased birth length, and increased weight

59. _____ usage during pregnancy may result in a shortened gestation and a higher incidence of fetal growth restriction.
   a. Cocaine
   b. Tobacco
   c. Alcohol
   d. Methamphetamine

Maternal Infections

60. The TORCH is a test used to detect maternal infection that may be teratogenic. Briefly explain this acronym.

61. An agent that produces congenital malformations or increases their incidence is called a(n)

   _____. List at least 3 of the most recognized drugs (chemical agents) for treating this agent.

Inborn Errors of Metabolism

62. Which of the following diseases is characterized by a deficiency in the hepatic enzyme phenylalanine hydroxylase?
    a. Tyrosine
    b. Phenylketonuria (PKU)
    c. Galactosemia
    d. Congenital hypothyroidism

63. What is the most common test for screening newborns for PKU?
    a. Guthrie blood test
    b. GeneTest
    c. Direct Coombs test
    d. Direct antiglobulin test

64. Identify the disorder in which galactose accumulates in the blood, inadvertently affecting several body organs. This includes hepatic dysfunction leading to cirrhosis, which results in jaundice in the infant by the second week of life.

APPLYING CRITICAL THINKING TO THE NURSING PRACTICE

A. Baby Abigail is admitted to the newborn nursery after an uncomplicated vertex delivery. During the initial assessment, the nurse notes a caput succedaneum over the left frontal area of Abigail's head.
   1. Differentiate between the following two types of head trauma that can occur during the birth process. Include information that the nurse would use to describe the injury to Abigail's parents.
      a. Caput succedaneum

      b. Cephalhematoma

   2. Early detection of a subgaleal hemorrhage is important. Identify the various ways a nurse can detect this hemorrhage on assessment.

B. The nurse is providing developmental care for a high-risk infant.
   1. What does a developmental approach for feeding the high-risk infant include?

   2. What does a developmental approach for conservation of energy include?

   3. What sleeping position is best for preterm infants, and why is this position best for them? How can the nurse prepare the infant and family to alter this position before discharge?

4. List at least four developmental interventions the nurse can include in the care plan.
   a.

   b.

   c.

   d.

C. The nurse is caring for a neonate who is receiving phototherapy.
   1. What two factors are primarily responsible for the development of physiologic jaundice in the newborn?
      a.

      b.

   2. How soon after birth would the nurse expect the following phases of physiologic jaundice to occur in the full-term infant?
      a. Onset

      b. Peak

      c. Plateau

   3. Identify the nursing interventions associated with the care of a child receiving phototherapy.
      a.

      b.

      c.

      d.

      e.

   4. Identify three potential negative effects related to parent-infant interaction in the infant receiving phototherapy.
      a.

      b.

      c.

D. Mandy is a premature infant in the intensive care unit. She has recovered from her respiratory distress and has been diagnosed as having an intraventricular hemorrhage. She is suspected of having sepsis.

 1. Postnatally, how might Mandy have obtained her infection?

 2. What clinical signs and symptoms suggest sepsis?

 3. What is the most important nursing goal for Mandy?

E. Mitch is a 3-day-old infant born to a mother who developed diabetes during pregnancy. Mitch was admitted to the NICU for observation.

 1. What is a common occurrence in infants of mothers with diabetes, and why?

 2. Why are early feedings of infants born to mothers with diabetes so important?

 3. What birth injuries are more common for the very large infant of a mother with diabetes?
    a.

    b.

    c.

9 | Health Promotion of the Infant and Family

Chapter 9 explores infancy, which is described as the period of development that has the fastest gain in physical size and the most dramatic developmental achievements. The biologic, psychosocial, cognitive, developmental, and social developments during the first year of life are presented. Factors related to temperament, concerns with parenting, and issues related to normal growth and development are also addressed. After completing this chapter, the student will be better prepared to provide nursing care that promotes optimal development in the infant and family.

REVIEW OF ESSENTIAL CONCEPTS

Promoting Optimal Growth and Development

1. John is a healthy infant who was born at a weight of 3.5 kg (7.7 pounds) and a height of 51 cm (20 inches). What will John's approximate weight and height be at 6 months of age?

2. Identify three factors that predispose the infant to more severe and acute respiratory problems.
   a.

   b.

   c.

3. At what age do maternal-derived iron stores begin to diminish in the infant?

4. What is the most immature of all the gastrointestinal organs throughout infancy?

5. List two reasons infants are susceptible to dehydration.
   a.

   b.

6. At what month of age are the hands predominantly closed, and what month of age are they are mostly open?

7. Which of the following abilities best describes the fine motor development of a normal 6-month-old?
    a. Can transfer objects from one hand to the other
    b. Can use one hand for grasping
    c. Can hold a cube in each hand simultaneously
    d. Can feed him- or herself a cracker

8. By what month of age is head control well established?

9. The infant is in Erikson's stage of developing a sense of trust. What are the crucial elements for achievement of this task?

10. The infant (birth to 24 months) is in what cognitive development stage, according to Piaget?

11. What three crucial events take place during the sensorimotor phase, when infants progress from reflexive behaviors to simple repetitive acts to imitative activity?
    a.

    b.

    c.

12. What disorder is a psychologic and developmental problem in which the infant may fail to seek and respond to comfort when distressed and may exhibit emotional dysregulation such as irritability?

13. Separation anxiety begins between what months, when the infant progresses through the first stage of separation-individuation and begins to have some awareness of self and mother as separate beings?

14. What is the infant's first means of verbal communication?

15. At what age can an infant ascribe meaning to a word?

16. What two important factors must be provided to the infant to achieve optimum social, emotional, and intellectual development?

    a.

    b.

17. Indicate whether each of the following statements is true or false.
    a. **T F** The type of toys given to the child is much less important than the quality of personal interaction that occurs.
    b. **T F** An increased risk of otitis media is associated with the use of a pacifier.
    c. **T F** The more harmony between the child's temperament and the parent's ability to accept and deal with the behavior, the greater the risk for subsequent parent-child conflicts.
    d. **T F** Infants innately explore during this phase of development, and parents need to take extra precautions in safeguarding the home.
    e. **T F** Pacifier use may have a protective effect on reducing the incidence of sudden infant death syndrome.

Promoting Optimal Health During Infancy

18. What mineral is human milk deficient in after the infant turns 6 months of age?

19. Expressed breast milk can be safely stored in the refrigerator for up to _____ day(s) without the risk of bacterial contamination.

20. When is it okay to introduce whole cow's milk to an infant?

21. Identify and offer a rationale for the first solid food introduced into the infant's diet.

22. What four elements need to be in place before introducing solid food to an infant?

    a.

    b.

    c.

    d.

23. Indicate whether each of the following statements is true or false.
    a. **T F** Active infants typically sleep less than placid infants.
    b. **T F** The American Academy of Pediatrics recommends all infants receive a daily supplement of vitamin C.
    c. **T F** Infants who are teething often have fever (>39° C), vomiting, and diarrhea.
    d. **T F** Iron supplements should be administered with whole cow's milk or milk products for greater absorption.

24. In order to identify food allergies, new food items are introduced to infants in what intervals?

25. Identify the three leading causes of accidental death injury in infants.

    a.

    b.

    c.

26. What is the most common cause of unintentional injuries resulting in emergency department visits among infants?

27. When driving a vehicle, the safest place for an infant is in the _____ seat.

APPLYING CRITICAL THINKING TO THE NURSING PRACTICE

A. Dean is a 6-month-old infant who is at the clinic for his checkup with his mother, Tami.
   1. What should the nurse assess regarding Dean's development behaviors of the attachment process?
      a.

      b.

      c.

d.

e.

2. What education can the nurse provide to Tami to enhance Dean's attachment to other family members?

B. Beverly is a 4-month-old infant in for a routine checkup. The nurse is providing anticipatory guidance to her mother, Becky, and father, John, on what they can expect over the next 2 months.
   1. List seven guidelines the nurse should give Becky and John related to starting Beverly on solid foods.
      a.

      b.

      c.

      d.

      e.

      f.

      g.

   2. The nurse stresses that the introduction of solid foods into Beverly's diet at this age is primarily for taste and chewing experience. Becky and John ask why that is the case. How should the nurse respond?

   3. Becky and John anticipate that Beverly will be teething soon and ask the nurse for information on comfort measures. How should the nurse respond?

C. The nurse is responsible for educating parents of 8- to 12-month-old infants on how to prevent accidental injury to their child.
   1. Identify at least five developmental characteristics the nurse assesses in the 8- to 12-month-old infant that predispose him or her to injury.
      a.

      b.

c.

d.

e.

2. What interventions can the nurse suggest to prevent burns in the child?
   a.

   b.

   c.

   d.

   e.

   f.

   g.

   h.

   i.

   j.

3. Why is choking still such a problem in this age group?

4. What is the rationale for not leaving medications in purses or handbags?

5. What steps can be taken to ensure safety of an infant in a home with a swimming pool?

10 Health Problems of Infants

Chapter 10 introduces common health problems of the first year of life, including nutritional disorders, feeding difficulties (eg, colic), growth failure, and sudden infant death syndrome (SIDS). After completing this chapter, the student will have the knowledge to provide adequate family-centered nursing care to infants who have these specific health problems.

REVIEW OF ESSENTIAL CONCEPTS

Nutritional Disorders

1. Identify five populations at risk for vitamin D deficiency, or rickets.

    a.

    b.

    c.

    d.

    e.

2. An excessive dose of a vitamin is generally defined as how many more times the recommended dietary allowance?

3. What vitamin supplement to prevent neural tube defects is recommended for all women of childbearing age? What is the daily recommended dose?

4. Low levels of zinc can cause what condition?

5. An imbalance in the intake of calcium and phosphorous may occur in infants who are given what instead of infant formula?

6. Children receiving high doses of what may have impaired vitamin C storage?

7. Hypervitaminosis of A and D presents the greatest problems because these _____ vitamins are stored in the body.

8. What vitamin supplement is recommended if the breastfeeding mother's intake of the vitamin is inadequate or if she is not taking vitamin supplements?

9. Malnutrition is a major health problem in the world for children under 5 years of age. What are the two major causes of this problem?
   a.

   b.

10. In the United States, severe protein and energy malnutrition are seen in children and adolescents with specific chronic health problems. Provide some examples of these illnesses or diseases.

11. Describe the appearance of a child with kwashiorkor.

12. _____ is a common occurrence in underdeveloped countries during times of drought, especially in cultures where adults eat first; the remaining food is often insufficient in quality and quantity for the children.

13. Identify the three management goals in treating protein and energy malnutrition that occurs as a result of persistent diarrhea.
    a.

    b.

    c.

14. Children who have one parent with a food allergy have a _____% greater risk of developing the allergy.

15. In most children, anaphylactic food reactions do not begin with skin signs, such as hives, red rash, and flushing. Rather, the reactions mimic what condition?

16. What three things should children with extremely sensitive food allergies do to ensure their safety?
   a.

   b.

   c.

17. What is considered the gold standard for diagnosing food allergies such as cow's milk allergy?

Feeding Difficulties
18. Define *colic*.

19. List nine elements of the nursing assessment that would be noted regarding colic.
   a.

   b.

   c.

   d.

   e.

   f.

   g.

h.

i.

20. Once the diagnosis of colic is established, what is the most important nursing intervention?

21. How do nurses play a critical role in the diagnosis of failure to thrive?

Growth Failure

22. What is the primary management of failure to thrive?

23. Identify at least three reasons that parents of infants with failure to thrive are at increased risk for attachment problems.

24. To prevent plagiocephaly, nurses should teach parents to place the infant in what position when awake?

Sudden Infant Death Syndrome

25. To prevent SIDS, the American Academy of Pediatrics recommends that healthy infants be placed in the

_____ position to sleep.

26. What groups of infants are at increased risk for SIDS?

27. What should the nurse avoid saying to parents after a SIDS death?

28. Some studies have found that _____ in infants is a protective factor against the occurrence of SIDS.

29. The most widely used monitoring for infants suspected of apnea is the _____.

30. The decision to discontinue home monitoring is based on what factors?

31. What three safety measures should the nurse discuss with parents of an infant being monitored at home for apnea?
   a.

   b.

   c.

APPLYING CRITICAL THINKING TO THE NURSING PRACTICE

A. Katie, age 16 years, comes into the emergency department with her parents. Katie has broken out in a red, itchy, raised rash over her face, chest, and upper outer thighs. On taking a detailed history, the nurse discovers Katie has recently eaten strawberry shortcake. Her tongue was swelling up and she was complaining of difficulty breathing, so her parents brought her in to the emergency department.
   1. Differentiate between a food allergy and food intolerance.

   2. Did Katie have a reaction that would be classified as a food allergy or food intolerance?

B. Don and Helen have brought in Kalen, their 2-month-old infant, to see the pediatrician. The parents' chief complaint is that for the past 3 weeks, Kalen has been having loud crying spells that last 4 hours a day. The parents report that Kalen draws his legs up to his abdomen while crying. On further examination, the nurse notes that he is tolerating breast milk and growing at a normal rate for his age.
   1. After reviewing the assessment data, the nurse determines that the infant may have colic on the basis of which symptoms?

2. What interventions can the nurse offer that might help with the colic symptoms?

C. Tommy, a 1-month-old infant, is admitted to the hospital for a diagnostic workup for apnea of infancy. Tommy's parents called the pediatrician when they noticed periods during which he stopped breathing and turned "blue."

1. Why is equipment safety a major area of nursing education if the infant is to be monitored at home?

2. What is the rationale for informing the local utility company and rescue squad of the home monitoring?

3. It must be stressed that monitors are only effective if they are _____ and there is a

_____ to alarms.

11 Health Promotion of the Toddler and Family

Chapter 11 presents issues relevant to the toddler period of development. The chapter highlights biologic, psychosocial, social, cognitive, and spiritual development during toddlerhood. Body image, gender identity, and coping with concerns related to normal growth and development are presented. At the completion of this chapter, the student will have the foundation to promote health and to meet the toddler's growth and development needs.

REVIEW OF ESSENTIAL CONCEPTS

Promoting Optimal Growth and Development

1. What period of time defines toddlerhood?

2. The growth rate slows considerably during the toddler years, and the birth weight is quadrupled by what years of age?

3. **T F** Chest circumference continues to increase in size and exceeds head circumference during the toddler years.

4. **T F** The toddler has a less well-developed abdominal musculature and short legs, giving him or her a pot-bellied appearance.

5. **T F** The respiratory rate, heart rate, and blood pressure increase during the toddler years.

6. One of the most prominent changes in the gastrointestinal system during the toddler period is the voluntary control

   of _____.

7. The physiologic ability to control the sphincters probably occurs between what age?

8. Identify the seven major psychosocial developmental tasks that must be dealt with during the toddler years.
   a.

   b.

   c.

   d.

e.

f.

g.

9. What is the developmental task of toddlerhood, according to Erikson?

10. Differentiate between negativism and ritualism, which are two characteristics typical of toddlers in their quest for autonomy.

11. According to Erikson, when the child can delay gratification, he or she has developed the _____.

12. How does Piaget describe the stage a 23-month-old child is in?

13. Describe Piaget's preoperational stage.

14. What factors strongly influence a child's perception of the world, including spirituality?

15. At what age can children refer to themselves by name?

16. Gender identity is developed by what age?

17. Describe the two phases of the toddler's task of differentiation of self from significant others.
    a. Separation

    b. Individuation

18. _____ is when the toddler separates from the mother and begins to make sense of experiences in the environment and then is drawn back to the mother for assistance in identifying the meaning of the experiences.

19. The typical child of 2 years has a vocabulary of approximately how many words, and approximately what percent of this speech is understandable?

20. What are some signs of independence in 15-month-old children?

21. Describe the type of play in which toddlers engage.

22. **T   F**   Bowel training is usually accomplished before bladder training in the toddler.

23. Identify the four markers that signal a child's readiness to toilet train.
    a.

    b.

    c.

    d.

24. When is a good time to start talking to a toddler about the addition of a new sibling to the family?

Chapter **11**   **Health Promotion of the Toddler and Family**

25. To minimize sibling rivalry, the parents should _____ the toddler in caregiving activities.

26. What are the best approaches for tapering temper tantrums?

27. What is one way in which parents can deal with negativism?

Promoting Optimal Health During Toddlerhood

28. What phenomenon refers to the toddler's decreased nutritional requirements and decreased appetite?

29. An appropriate way to determine adequate serving size for a toddler is to give _____ of solid food for each year of age.

30. What are the most effective ways to remove plaque from teeth?

31. How much toothpaste should be used for toddlers?

32. When do toothbrushes need to be replaced?

33. What is the cause of most accidental deaths in all pediatric age groups after age 1 year?

34. Toddlers up to 24 months of age are safer riding in convertible seats in what position?

35. Children should use specially designed car restraints until they are 145 cm (4 feet, 9 inches) in height and are how old?

36. What is the most common type of thermal injury in children?

37. What is the major reason for accidental poisoning in young children?

APPLYING CRITICAL THINKING TO THE NURSING PRACTICE

A. A young mother brings her 2-year-old son, Greg, into a well-child clinic for a routine checkup. Height and weight are obtained; the child's height is 89 cm (35 inches), and his weight is 13.6 kg (30 pounds).
   1. Plot Greg's height and weight on a growth chart. How do his measurements compare with norms for this age?
      a. Height

      b. Weight

   2. Greg's mother is concerned because he has gained only 2 pounds and grown 2 inches since his 20-month checkup. What information does the nurse need to give this mother regarding healthy toddler development?

   3. Identify three developmental milestones that Greg should have accomplished in the following areas:
      a. Gross motor development

      b. Fine motor development

      c. Language development

   4. Greg's mother describes his play activity as, "He plays near others his age but makes no attempt to play or interact with them." How should the nurse respond to this comment?

5. What information can the nurse relay to Greg's mother on selecting appropriate play activities for him?
   a.

   b.

6. Greg is not yet toilet-trained, but he is showing signs of interest in flushing the toilet and asking questions about the potty. His mother asks when she should begin trying to train him. Which of the following is the best response the nurse can give this mother?
   a. Greg will need to be able to sit on the toilet for 10 to 15 minutes at a time.
   b. A factor in successful training is the child's desire to please the mother by controlling impulses to defecate and urinate.
   c. Bladder training should be attempted first, since the child usually has a stronger and more regular urge to urinate.
   d. Attempts to begin toilet training before age 3 are usually unsuccessful because myelinization of the spinal cord is incomplete.

7. Greg's mother asks questions about dental care. The nurse describes the following conditions that can lead to early childhood caries (ECC) for a toddler:
   a.

   b.

   c.

   d.

B. Interview the parents of a toddler about typical toddler behaviors (eg, negativism, management of temper tantrums, and eating and sleep patterns). Answer the following questions, including specific interventions associated with these issues.
   1. How is negativism most often manifested in the toddler? How can this manifestation be decreased?

   2. How does negativism contribute to the toddler's acquisition of a sense of autonomy?

   3. Why are temper tantrums so prevalent in the toddler age group?

4. Identify four eating behaviors that are characteristic of toddlers.

    a.

    b.

    c.

    d.

5. Why is nutritional counseling for parents with toddlers an important nursing intervention?

6. Sleep problems are common in this age group. The problems are most likely related to what types of fears?

7. What three interventions can a parent use to reduce toddler sleep problems?

    a.

    b.

    c.

C. You are going on a routine visit with a home health care nurse. Assess the home of a toddler for the presence of potential safety hazards. Answer the following questions.

1. What are the two key determinants that can reduce the number of unintentional childhood injuries with catastrophic results?

    a.

    b.

2. Why is there a critical increase in injuries during the toddler years?

3. What categories of injuries are common during the toddler years?

    a.

    b.

c.

d.

e.

f.

g.

4. What five factors could pose a safety hazard to a toddler in the home?

   a.

   b.

   c.

   d.

   e.

5. Match the following developmental accomplishments with the appropriate safety measures. (Answers may be used more than once.)

   a. _____ Walks, runs, climbs

   b. _____ Exhibits curiosity

   c. _____ Pulls objects

   d. _____ Puts things in mouth

   1. Closely supervise when toddler is near a source of water.
   2. Choose toys without removable parts.
   3. Turn pot handles toward the back of the stove.
   4. Place all toxic agents out of reach in a locked cabinet.
   5. Place child-protector caps on all medicines and poisons.
   6. Cover electrical outlets with protective plastic caps.
   7. Avoid giving sharp or pointed objects to the toddler.
   8. Keep hanging tablecloths out of toddler's reach.
   9. Lock fences and doors if toddlers are not directly supervised.

12 Health Promotion of the Preschooler and Family

Chapter 12 focuses on the development of the child in the preschool period, which is the most critical period of emotional and psychologic development. The chapter discusses biologic, cognitive, psychosocial, moral, and spiritual development of the preschooler and family. Issues related to body image, sexuality, and normal growth and development are outlined. The chapter provides the student with information for promoting optimal health during the preschool years and introduces areas of special concern for parents and family members. This knowledge will enable the student to develop nursing goals and interventions that foster the normal development of the preschooler and that assist parents in coping with the associated developmental difficulties.

REVIEW OF ESSENTIAL CONCEPTS

Promoting Optimal Growth and Development

1. The rate of physical growth _____ and _____ during the preschool years.

2. **T   F**   Preschoolers maintain the pot-bellied appearance of the toddler.

3. **T   F**   During the preschool period, the separation-individuation process is completed.

4. By what year of age, can the child skip on alternate feet, jump rope, and begin to skate and swim?

5. According to Erikson, the chief psychosocial task of the preschool period is acquiring a sense of what? Conflict arises when preschoolers experience what?

6. What two cognitive tasks are related to the preschool period?
   a.

   b.

7. Piaget's preoperational phase consists of which two phases?
   a.

   b.

8. According to Piaget, what method becomes the child's way of understanding, adjusting to, and working out life's experiences?

9. **T   F**   Preschoolers increasingly use language without comprehending the meaning of words, particularly concepts of right and left, causality, and time.

10. Describe how preschoolers use causality and give an example.

11. Preschoolers' thinking is often magical. What does this mean?

12. **T   F**   In preschoolers' minds, calling them bad means they are bad persons.

13. Development of the _____ is strongly linked to spiritual development.

14. **T   F**   During the preschool years, vocabulary increases dramatically.

15. Why are bandages critical to the preschooler who has just had abdominal surgery?

16. Preschoolers are forming strong attachments to the _____ parent while identifying with the

    _____ parent.

17. An average child can be expected to have a vocabulary of how many words by the age of 6 years?

18. Contrast language development in 3- to 4-year-old children with language development in 4- to 5-year-old children.

19. Describe the type of play most apparent during the preschool years.

20. Identify three functions served by imaginary playmates.

    a.

    b.

    c.

21. There are no absolute indicators for school readiness, but what factors are important to consider?

22. List three opportunities that preschools or daycare centers provide for children.

    a.

    b.

    c.

23. What factor is recommended when evaluating a preschool or daycare center?

24. Identify the two rules that govern answering a child's questions about sex or other sensitive issues.

    a.

    b.

25. What is a normal part of sexual curiosity and exploration for the preschooler?

26. What are some of the preschool child's most common fears?

    a.

    b.

c.

d.

e.

f.

27. What is the best way to help children overcome their fears?

28. Why are young children especially vulnerable to stress?

29. Identify the five factors that differentiate "problematic" aggression from "normal" aggression.
    a.

    b.

    c.

    d.

    e.

30. The most critical period for speech development occurs between what years of age?

31. The failure to master sensorimotor integrations results in what during the preschool years? Is this finding more frequent in boys or girls?

32. **T F**   The Denver Articulation Screening Examination is an excellent tool for assessing a child's articulation skills.

Promoting Optimal Health During the Preschool Years

33. Protein requirements increase with age. What is the recommended intake for preschoolers?

34. According to MyPlate, how many servings of fruits and vegetables should a child receive daily?

35. Excessive consumption of what has been associated with dental caries?

36. **T F**   The quality of the food consumed is more important than the quantity.

37. **T F**   Although preschoolers' fine motor control is improved, they still require assistance and supervision with brushing, and flossing should be performed by parents.

38. **T F**   During the preschool years, the emphasis in injury prevention is placed on education for safety and potential hazards to prevent injury.

APPLYING CRITICAL THINKING TO THE NURSING PRACTICE

A. Thom, a 5-year-old boy, is brought to the pediatrician's office by his mother for a well-child visit. During the assessment, the nurse finds that Thom is 106.7 cm (42 inches) tall and weighs 17.7 kg (39 pounds).
   1. Plot Thom's height and weight on a growth chart. How do his measurements compare with the norms for this age?
      a. Height

      b. Weight

   2. What factors should the nurse include in the teaching plan regarding the physical growth of a preschooler?

   3. Before the physical examination, the nurse questions Thom's mother about his developmental progress. Identify three developmental milestones that Thom should have accomplished in the following areas:
      a. Gross motor development

      b. Fine motor development

      c. Language development

Chapter **12**   **Health Promotion of the Preschooler and Family**

4. Thom has had an imaginary friend, named "Boy," since he turned 3 years old. His mother is beginning to wonder whether "Boy" will be with Thom forever. What information should the nurse give Thom's mother regarding imaginary friends?

5. What types of toys, playthings, and activities could be recommended to foster Thom's development in each of the following areas?
   a. Physical play

   b. Dramatic play

6. How could the nurse guide Thom's mother on family-centered care during the preschool years?

B. Sydney, a 5-year-old girl, and her parents are in for a well-child checkup. The nurse is interviewing her parents. The interview reveals that Sydney is attending a preschool program. Answer the following questions and include specific responses to illustrate these concepts.
   1. What does the nurse identify as the most important aspect of a preschool or daycare program?

   2. List the some of the factors Sydney's parents should assess in the preschool or daycare.
      a.

      b.

      c.

      d.

      e.

      f.

      g.

3. The nurse questions Sydney's parents on how they prepared Sydney for preschool. Identify four ways parents should prepare children for preschool.

a.

b.

c.

d.

C. Answer the following questions about sex education, sleep disturbances, dental health, and eating patterns and include specific responses to illustrate these concepts.

1. Why is preschool age an appropriate time to begin sex education?

2. Identify why preschool years are a prime time for sleep disturbances.

3. How often should routine dental care by a dentist be provided to preschoolers?

4. A variety of health problems among adults are thought to be influenced by eating patterns established in the preschool years. What goal would you encourage parents to achieve related to the intake of fat in this age group?

5. What should parents be informed of regarding the intake of carbonated beverages in young children?

13 Health Problems of Toddlers and Preschoolers

Chapter 13 introduces nursing considerations essential to the care of the young child experiencing health problems. This chapter addresses a variety of topics, including infectious disorders, intestinal parasitic diseases, ingestion of injurious agents, and child maltreatment. After completing this chapter, the student will be prepared to develop nursing goals and interventions directed at assessing and managing health problems of toddlers and preschoolers, with the goal of achieving a state of optimum health.

REVIEW OF ESSENTIAL CONCEPTS

1. List six consequences of inadequate sleep in children.
    a.

    b.

    c.

    d.

    e.

    f.

2. _____ traditions may dictate sleep practices contrary to well-accepted professional recommendations.

3. Research has revealed a direct correlation between sleep problems in preschool children and what two factors?
    a.

    b.

4. What interventions can be recommended to parents for children who delay going to bed?
    a.

    b.

    c.

5. Differentiate between nightmares and sleep terrors.

6. _____ is an inflammatory reaction of the skin to chemical substances, natural or synthetic, that evokes a hypersensitivity response or direct irritation.

7. What is the major goal in the treatment of contact dermatitis?

8. What are the offending substances in poison oak, ivy, and sumac?

9. When it is known that the child has made contact with poison oak, ivy, or sumac, what immediate response should the nurse educate the family to implement?

10. What type of anthropod injects venom deadly enough to require immediate attention?

11. General wound care of animal bites consists of rinsing the wound with copious amounts of what solution?

12. Prophylactic antibiotics are indicated for what types of animal bites?

13. The most important aspect related to animal bites is _____.

14. Why do all human bites need immediate medical attention?

Chapter **13** **Health Problems of Toddlers and Preschoolers**

15. Hot-water scalds are most frequent in what age group?

16. What two factors are considered in assessing the severity of a burn?
    a.

    b.

17. Match the type of burn with the correct definition

    a. _____ Partial-thickness
       (second-degree)
       burn

    b. _____ Superficial
       (first-degree) burn

    c. _____ Fourth-degree burn

    d. _____ Full-thickness
       (third-degree) burn

    1. Minor burn involving the epidermal layer only; usually consist of a latent period followed by erythema
    2. Involves the epidermis and varying degrees of the dermis; painful, moist, red, and blistered
    3. Involves the muscle, fascia, and bone
    4. Involves the epidermis and dermis and extends into subcutaneous tissue; destroys nerve endings, sweat glands, and hair follicles

18. **T   F**   A burn that is 5% of the total body surface area can be life threatening if not treated correctly.

19. What are some of the clinical manifestations of an inhalation injury?

20. Following a serious thermal injury what is the immediate threat to life?

21. A less common complication of a thermal injury is _____, resulting from fluid overload or acute respiratory distress syndrome (ARDS) in association with gram-negative sepsis.

22. Indicate whether each of the following statements regarding emergency care of burns is true or false.
    a. **T   F**   It is helpful to place a wet dressing on a burn victim to enhance circulation to the burned area and decrease tissue damage.
    b. **T   F**   Chemical burns require continuous flushing with large amounts of water before transport to a medical facility.
    c. **T   F**   The use of neutralizing agents on the skin is contraindicated, because a chemical reaction is initiated and further injury may result.
    d. **T   F**   Burned clothing should be left in place to prevent further damage.

23. What immunization should be administered prophylactically to a burn patient if more than 5 years have passed since the last immunization?

24. List the six objectives of fluid therapy in the burn patient.

    a.

    b.

    c.

    d.

    e.

    f.

25. What type of intravenous solution is used during the initial phase of therapy for burn patients?

26. What type of diet is encouraged for the burn patient to provide adequate nutrition for healing?

27. What vitamins are administered in the early postburn period to facilitate growth and proliferation of epithelial cells?

28. What is the drug of choice for managing pain in burn victims?

29. Management of partial-thickness wounds requires _____ of devitalized tissue to promote healing.

30. Describe the purpose of hydrotherapy.

31. Match the skin coverings with the description.

   a. _____ Allograft (homograft)

   b. _____ Xenograft

   c. _____ Synthetic skin coverings

   d. _____ Sheet graft

   e. _____ Mesh graft

1. Composed of a variety of materials and is used for the management of partial-thickness burns and donor sites
2. Sheet of skin obtained from the donor site and passed through a mesher and is used in a less desirable area
3. Obtained from human cadavers and is used as a temporary skin covering of extensive burns
4. Obtained from a variety of species and is used when extensive early debridement is indicated to cover partial-thickness burns
5. Sheet of skin obtained from the donor site and is used in areas where cosmetic results are more visible

32. **T F** Education related to fire safety and survival among young children should include use of a fire extinguisher.

33. Treatment of sunburn involves what three factors?

   a.

   b.

   c.

34. If an individual normally burns in 10 minutes without sunscreen, use of a sunscreen with a sun protection factor of 15 allows the individual to remain in the sun for how long before acquiring the same degree of burn?

35. What action is recommended to parents if the exact quantity or type of ingested toxin is not known?

36. List the three principles of emergency treatment following the ingestion of toxic agents.

   a.

   b.

   c.

37. What is the first and most important principle in dealing with a poisoning?

38. _____ is no longer recommended for immediate treatment of poison ingestion.

39. Match the following poisoning with the correct antidote.

   a. _____ Acetaminophen poisoning

   b. _____ Carbon monoxide inhalation

   c. _____ Opioid overdose

   d. _____ Benzodiazepine overdose

   e. _____ Digoxin toxicity

   f. _____ Cyanide poisoning

   g. _____ Poisonous bites

   1. Oxygen
   2. *N*-acetylcysteine
   3. Flumazenil (Romazicon)
   4. Naloxone
   5. Digibind
   6. Amyl nitrate
   7. Antivenin

40. The most frequent source of acute childhood lead poisoning is deteriorating _____ in older homes or lead-contamination in the yard.

41. List the risk factors for having high blood lead levels.
   a.

   b.

   c.

   d.

42. What system is the more vulnerable for damage when young children are exposed to lead compared with older children and adults?

43. What test is used to determine the level of lead exposure?

44. What are some of the long-term neurocognitive signs of lead poisoning?

45. What is the primary nursing goal in lead poisoning?

46. In 2011, Child Protective Service agencies in the United States confirmed that an estimated _____ children were victims of child maltreatment.

47. What is the most common form of child maltreatment?

48. What are common internal findings in infants who have been violently shaken?

49. Define the term Munchausen syndrome by proxy (MSP).

50. **T   F**   Child maltreatment occurs most often in lower socioeconomic families.

51. What three risk factors are commonly identified in child abuse?
    a.

    b.

    c.

52. Identify five significant risk factors for child sexual abuse.
    a.

    b.

    c.

    d.

    e.

53. **T   F**   Cases of abuse are often detected by inconsistencies in the history of events given by the child or caregiver, with the history of events not matching physical findings.

A. Kim, a 3-year-old girl, comes to clinic for a routine checkup. Mom reports difficulty getting Kim to bed, then Kim has trouble going to sleep and often wakes during the night.
   1. What should be assessed as possible causes of these sleep problems?

   2. What interventions can the nurse teach to Kim's mom to minimize or eliminate Kim's sleep problems?

B. Mrs. Ryan brings 5-year-old Sean to the clinic because he has several patches over his legs and arms that are red, swollen, and itching. She reports he was out playing in a wooded area with his father 2 days previously. On examination, you discover that Sean has localized, streaked impetiginous lesions typically resulting from poison ivy, oak, or sumac.
   1. What is the treatment of choice?

   2. Identify three nursing interventions for teaching Sean's family how to immediately respond to this type of incident in the future.
      a.

      b.

      c.

C. Michael brought his 9-year-old son, James, to see the nurse practitioner. He complains that James has developed learning and behavior problems over the past year since they moved into town. Answer the following questions related to this scenario.
   1. What question could the nurse practitioner ask to assess James's level of possible contamination from lead exposure?

   2. What are some early signs of moderate- to low-dose exposure to lead?

   3. What does the nurse identify as the initial goal for children with low-level exposure to lead?

4. After James is tested, the results reveal he has an elevated blood lead level of 11 mcg/dl. What factors need to be included in the family-centered teaching plan related to the care of James?

D. Danny is a 2-year-old boy hospitalized as a result of maltreatment. He is a highly energetic boy. He is being raised by his mother, who has to work two full-time jobs to make ends meet. He is in the hospital because his mother hit him and locked him in the closet because she "just can't take it anymore." Answer the following questions related to this scenario.
   1. Identify characteristics in each of the following areas that can be used to assess the vulnerability of families, in general, to abuse.
      a. Parents

      b. Child

      c. Environment

   2. Identify at least five red flags that the nurse should link to possible abuse when obtaining a patient and family history.
      a.

      b.

      c.

      d.

      e.

   3. Develop three nursing diagnoses that could be used as a basis for the care of this family.
      a.

      b.

      c.

14 Health Promotion of the School-Age Child and Family

Chapter 14 discusses the school-age developmental stage, which is characterized by greater social awareness and social skills. Biologic, cognitive, psychosocial, moral, and spiritual development related to the school-age child and family is outlined. At the completion of this chapter, the student will be able to use knowledge of the school-age child's growth and development to formulate nursing goals and interventions that foster health promotion and maintenance behaviors in school-age children and their families.

REVIEW OF ESSENTIAL CONCEPTS

Promoting Optimal Growth and Development

1. Physiologically, the middle years begin with the shedding of the first _____ and end at

   puberty, with the acquisition of the _____.

2. **T   F**   During the school-age years, a child will grow approximately 5 cm (2 inches) per year and will almost triple in weight.

3. Identify the three most pronounced physiologic changes that indicate increasing maturity in the school-age child.
   a.

   b.

   c.

4. What is the average age of puberty for girls and boys?

5. According to Freud, the school-age child is in which of the following periods?
   a. Oral
   b. Anal
   c. Oedipal
   d. Latency

6. According to Erikson, the developmental task of middle childhood is acquiring a sense of which of the following?
   a. Trust
   b. Autonomy
   c. Initiative
   d. Industry

7. According to Erikson, failure to develop a sense of accomplishment results in a sense of _____.

8. **T   F**   Children with physical or mental limitations may be at a disadvantage for skill acquisition and are therefore at risk of feeling inferior.

9. According to Piaget, the school-age child is in which stage?
   a. Sensorimotor
   b. Preoperational
   c. Concrete operational
   d. Formal operational

10. According to Piaget, what occurs when children can recognize that changing the shape of a substance, such as a lump of clay, does not alter its total mass?

11. There is a developmental sequence in children's capacity to conserve matter. Conservation of _____

    is usually grasped before conservation of _____.

12. Define the term *classification*.

13. **T   F**   The most significant and valuable tool acquired during the school-age years is the ability to read.

14. Which of the following best describes the younger (6- to 7-year-old) school-age child's perception of rules and judgment of actions?
    a. Judges an act by its intentions rather than by the consequences alone
    b. Believes that rules and judgments are not absolute
    c. Understands the reasons behind rules
    d. Interprets accidents and misfortunes as punishments for misdeeds

15. Which of the following best describes the older (11- to 12-year-old) school-age child's perception of rules and judgment of actions?
    a. Does not understand the reasons for rules
    b. Takes into account different points of view to make a judgment
    c. Judges an act by its consequences
    d. Believes that rules and judgments are absolute

16. One of the most important socializing agents in the school-age years is the _____ group.

17. What has a strong influence on the child's attainment of independence from parents?

18. Identify three valuable lessons children learn from daily interactions with age-mates.
    a.

    b.

    c.

19. Poor relationships with peers and a lack of group identification can contribute to _____.

20. Where does bullying most frequently occur?

21. Team play teaches children to modify or exchange personal goals for goals of the group; it also teaches them that

_____ is an effective strategy for attaining a goal.

22. The term _____ refers to a conscious awareness of self-perceptions, such as one's physical characteristics, abilities, values, ideals, and expectations, as well as an idea of self in relation to others. It also includes one's body image, sexuality, and self-esteem.

23. **T   F**   School-age children are not prepared to abandon all parental control.

24. _____ serve as role models with whom children identify and whom they try to emulate.

25. Children who spend some amount of time before or after school without supervision of an adult are termed

_____.

26. Identify five factors that influence the amount and manner of discipline and limit-setting imposed on school-age children.
    a.

    b.

    c.

    d.

    e.

27. Identify eight signs of stress in school-age children.
    a.

    b.

    c.

    d.

Chapter **14** **Health Promotion of the School-Age Child and Family**

e.

f.

g.

h.

Promoting Optimal Health During the School Years

28. Match each behavior with the age at which it is typically exhibited.

a. _____ Develops concept of numbers

b. _____ Enjoys group activities involving own sex but is beginning
to mix with members of opposite sex

c. _____ Enjoys group sports and organizations

d. _____ Loves friends; talks incessantly about them

e. _____ Likes simple card games

1. 6 years
2. 9 years
3. 12 years

29. Several factors have been identified as contributing to childhood obesity. Name three of those factors.

a.

b.

c.

30. **T   F**   The appearance of permanent teeth in the school-age child begins with the eruption of the 6-year molar.

31. **T   F**   An important component of ongoing sex education is effective communication with parents.

32. **T   F**   School nurses are vital to the development, implementation, and evaluation of health care plans for
chronically ill or disabled children.

33. **T   F**   The most common cause of severe accidental injury and death in school-age children is poisoning.

A. Cole, age 9 years, is brought to the pediatrician's office by his mother, Ann, for his annual physical examination. His height is 132 cm (52 inches), and his weight is 28.1 kg (62 pounds). His vision is evaluated as 20/30 in both eyes.
1. Plot Cole's height and weight on a growth chart. How do his measurements compare with the norms for this age?
   a. Height

   b. Weight

2. Ann tells the nurse that Cole likes to help his father with the yard work. However, Cole's work is not always up to his father's expectations. What information about normal development could the nurse offer Ann?

3. Ann expresses concern because she is having a problem with dishonesty in her 6-year-old daughter. What information could the nurse provide to assist her in dealing with this concern?

B. A nurse interviews a school-age child and his or her parents about changing interpersonal relationships and peer groups. Answer the following questions and include specific responses to illustrate the concepts.
1. The parents ask the nurse why school-age children spend an increased amount of time away from their homes and families. What is the best response the nurse can offer this family?

2. The parents want to know why relationships with age-mates are so important in the life of the school-age child. What is the best response the nurse can offer this family?

3. What would the nurse include in a teaching plan for parents of a school-age child to prevent injury to the child from motor vehicle accidents?
   a.

   b.

   c.

   d.

   e.

4. What would the nurse include in a teaching plan for parents of a school-age child to prevent accidental drowning?

   a.

   b.

   c.

   d.

   e.

   f.

15 Health Promotion of the Adolescent and Family

Chapter 15 examines the adolescent period, which is a period of transition from childhood to adulthood. After completing this chapter, the student will understand the interplay of physical, psychosocial, and emotional factors in the adolescent's development and interpersonal relationships. This knowledge will enable the student to provide anticipatory guidance to assist the child and family with the intricate developmental issues of adolescence.

REVIEW OF ESSENTIAL CONCEPTS

Promoting Optimal Growth and Development

1. The term *adolescence* covers the ages of _____ to _____

   years, while the term *teenagers* describes ages _____ to _____
   years.

2. Define the following terms:
   a. Puberty

   b. Adolescence

3. What are the two most obvious physical changes that occur during adolescence?
   a.

   b.

4. _____ are the external and internal organs that carry out the reproductive functions (eg, ovaries, uterus, breasts, penis).

5. _____ are the changes that occur throughout the body as a result of hormonal changes (eg, voice alterations, development of facial and pubertal hair, fat deposits) but that play no direct part in reproduction.

6. _____ is the feminizing hormone, whereas _____ are the masculinizing hormones.

7. What assessment tool is used to determine sexual maturity level based on sex characteristics and genital development?

8. The normal age range for the onset of menarche is usually considered to be _____ to

   _____ years; the average age is _____.

9. The first pubescent changes in boys are _____ enlargement and the initial appearance of

_____.

10. Hormonal activity during puberty is controlled by the _____ in response to a stimulus

from the _____.

11. _____ are responsible for the development of pubic, axillary, and body hair; acne; body
odor; and height increase.

12. **T   F**   Enlargement of the larynx and vocal cords occurs in both boys and girls to produce voice changes.

13. **T   F**   The size and strength of the heart, blood volume, systolic blood pressure, pulse rate, respiratory rate, and
basal metabolic rate all increase during adolescence.

14. What is the developmental task of adolescence, according to Erikson?

15. A sense of _____ identity appears to be an essential precursor to the sense of personal
identity.

16. Why are adolescents frequently labeled as unstable, inconsistent, and unpredictable?

17. According to Piaget, adolescents are no longer restricted to the real and actual, which was typical of the period of
concrete thought; now they are concerned with the possible and can think beyond the present. What does Piaget call
this stage of development?

18. Identify five characteristics that are typical of the adolescent's thought processes.
    a.

    b.

    c.

    d.

    e.

19. Which has more influence on an adolescent's self-evaluation and behavior: peer group or parents?

20. Greater levels of _____ and _____ are associated with fewer high-risk behaviors and more health-promoting behaviors.

21. Define *authoritative parenting*.

22. What adolescent behaviors has parental monitoring been found to directly influence?

23. **T F** Adolescents prefer to bring up the subject of sex to the health care provider rather than having the health care provider broach the subject.

24. **T F** Sexuality in middle adolescence involves internal identification of heterosexual, homosexual, or bisexual attractions.

25. **T F** It has been determined that the body image established during late adolescence is temporary and subject to change.

Promoting Optimal Health During Adolescence

26. Identify seven causes of morbidity in adolescence.
    a.

    b.

    c.

    d.

    e.

    f.

    g.

27. **T F** The increase in height, weight, muscle mass, and sexual maturity of adolescence is accompanied by greater nutritional requirements.

28. What are two major contributing factors to the increase in both children and adolescent obesity in the United States?

a.

b.

29. Routine nutrition screening for adolescents should include questions about what topics?

30. To have improved health outcomes, school-age children and adolescents should engage in how many minutes or more of moderate to vigorous physical activity daily?

31. Identify five major areas of stress for the adolescent.

a.

b.

c.

d.

e.

32. **T F** The long-term effects of tanning include premature aging of the skin; increased risk of skin cancer; and, in susceptible individuals, phototoxic reactions.

33. **T F** Suicide is the greatest single cause of death in the adolescent age group.

34. **T F** The use of alcohol, driving too fast, and using a cell phone to talk or text are contributing factors for fatal and nonfatal motor vehicle accidents in teenagers.

APPLYING CRITICAL THINKING TO THE NURSING PRACTICE

A. Britney is a 14-year-old girl who comes to the pediatric clinic for a yearly checkup. She is accompanied by her mother. Britney appears overweight and has noticeable acne on her face and forehead. Her age of menarche was 1 year ago.

1. Britney's height is 162.6 cm (64 inches), and her weight is 73 kg (161 pounds). How do her measurements compare with those of other girls her age?

a. Height

b. Weight

2. What principles related to adolescent growth and hormonal changes should be explained to Britney, since she is concerned about her weight and acne?

B. Billy, age 16, came into the physician's office for an annual physical examination. His mother, Kim, is concerned because he has recently developed a lack of interest in family activities and prefers to "hang out" with his buddies from school. Answer the following questions on how the nurse can provide education on normal adolescent behaviors and stages to Kim.

1. How could the nurse explain to Kim the role of the peer group in the development of adolescent identity?

2. What specific examples could the nurse give Kim on how group identity is demonstrated by the adolescent?

3. Kim asks the nurse why peer groups are so important during the adolescent years. What is the nurse's best response to her question?

C. Interview an adolescent about his health promotion behavior. Answer the following questions and include specific responses to illustrate these concepts.

1. Why might adolescents complain of fatigue?

2. What positive benefits come from participation in sports?

3. What developmental characteristics predispose the adolescent to accidents?

Chapter **15** **Health Promotion of the Adolescent and Family**

16 Health Problems of School-Age Children and Adolescents

Chapter 16 details common health problems and situations that are integral to the care of the school-age child and the adolescent. This chapter introduces students to concepts needed in the care of school-age children and adolescents with altered growth and maturation, issues related to sexuality, and a variety of other health problems.

REVIEW OF ESSENTIAL CONCEPTS

Problems Related to Elimination

1. _____ is a common and troublesome disorder that is defined as intentional or involuntary passage of urine into bed (usually at night) in children who are beyond the age when voluntary bladder control should normally have been acquired.

2. List the various therapeutic techniques that can be employed to manage enuresis.
   a.

   b.

   c.

   d.

   e.

   f.

3. **T   F**   Punishment for bed-wetting is a successful way to reduce its occurrence.

4. _____ is the repeated voluntary or involuntary passage of feces of normal or near-normal consistency into places not appropriate for that purpose according to the individual's own sociocultural setting.

5. What is one of the most common causes of encopresis?

6. _____ is soiling caused by emotional problems.

7. Enuresis is more common in _____; nocturnal bed-wetting usually ceases between

_____ and _____ years of age.

8. A bladder volume of _____ to _____ ml (10–12 ounces) is sufficient to hold a night's urine.

Disorders Related to the Reproductive System

9. Define the two types of amenorrhea.
   a. Primary

   b. Secondary

10. The treatment of choice for dysmenorrhea in adolescents is the administration of nonsteroidal antiinflammatory

    drugs, which block the formation of _____.

11. _____ is important in the prevention and management of vaginal discharge.

12. List the symptoms of premenstrual syndrome.

13. What strategies can significantly improve premenstrual syndrome symptoms and are encouraged before recommending medicines?

Health Problems Related to Sexuality

14. Identify three factors that have contributed to the downward trend of adolescent pregnancy rates in the United States.
    a.

    b.

    c.

15. Medical concerns of pregnant adolescents include:
    a.

    b.

    c.

16. What is one of the greatest dangers adolescents face with unprotected sexual activity?

17. Differentiate between primary and secondary prevention of sexually transmitted infections in adolescents.

18. Match the following sexually transmitted infections with their causative organisms and the drug of choice for treatment.

a. _____ Gonorrhea

b. _____ Chlamydial infection

c. _____ Herpes progenitalis

d. _____ Syphilis

e. _____ Trichomoniasis

1. *C. trachomatis*
2. Herpes simplex virus (HSV)
3. *Trichomonas vaginalis*
4. *Neisseria gonorrhoeae*
5. *Treponema pallidum*
6. Metronidazole
7. Doxycycline
8. Acyclovir
9. Penicillin
10. Ceftriaxone

19. **T   F**   Infertility is a long-term effect of pelvic inflammatory disease.

20. Identify the presenting symptoms of pelvic inflammatory disease.

21. **T   F**   Acquaintance rape is far more common than stranger rape.

22. **T   F**   Rape victims need to know that they are all right and are not being blamed for the situation.

23. **T   F**   The primary goal of nursing care for the rape victim is to get every detail of the rape, even if the patient is overwhelmed.

Eating Disorders

24. What measurement is recommended as the most accurate method for screening children and adolescents for obesity?

25. What eight health conditions are related to childhood and adolescent obesity?
    a.

    b.

    c.

    d.

    e.

116

f.

g.

h.

26. What results from a caloric intake that consistently exceeds caloric requirements and expenditure?

27. Which race/ethnicity among adolescents is at greatest risk for overweight and obesity?

28. **T F** For the first time in U.S. history, the current generation of children will have a shorter life expectancy than their parents.

29. **T F** The best approach to the management of obesity is preventive.

30. **T F** Diet modification is an essential part of weight reduction.

31. Define *anorexia nervosa*.

32. Identify five typical characteristics of individuals with anorexia nervosa.
    a.

    b.

    c.

    d.

33. List eight clinical manifestations of anorexia nervosa.
    a.

    b.

c.

d.

e.

f.

g.

h.

34. List six family characteristics associated with eating disorders.
    a.

    b.

    c.

    d.

    e.

    f.

35. Define *bulimia*.

36. Define *binge eating disorder*.

37. **T**　**F**　The female athlete triad refers to young women with eating disorders, excessive exercising, and low heart rate.

38. List the two most important goals for patients with anorexia nervosa.

    a.

    b.

39. How can refeeding syndrome be avoided?

Disorders with Behavioral Components

40. Define *attention deficit hyperactivity disorder (ADHD)*.

41. What conditions should be ruled out before a diagnosis of ADHD is made?

42. List the five components of the multifactorial approach to the management of ADHD.

    a.

    b.

    c.

    d.

    e.

43. **T   F**   Posttraumatic stress disorder (PTSD) refers to the development of characteristic symptoms after exposure to an extremely traumatic experience or catastrophic event.

44. **T   F**   Causes of PTSD can include automobile, school, or recreational accidents or bullying.

45. **T   F**   A striking feature of school phobia is the prompt subsiding of symptoms when it is evident that the child can remain at home.

46. **T   F**   A primary goal for treating school phobia is encouraging the child to keep up with schoolwork.

Chapter **16   Health Problems of School-Age Children and Adolescents**

47. Define *conversion reaction.*

48. Why is depression often difficult to detect in children?

49. List the seven behavioral characteristics of children with depression.
    a.

    b.

    c.

    d.

    e.

    f.

    g.

50. **T   F**   The basic disturbance in childhood schizophrenia is a lack of contact with reality and the subsequent development of a world of the child's own.

Serious Health Problems of Later Childhood and Adolescence

51. Why do adolescents begin to smoke?

52. **T   F**   Smoking-prevention programs that focus on the negative, long-term effects of smoking on health have been effective.

53. What are the two broad categories of adolescents who use drugs?
    a.

    b.

54. What are the most notable effects of alcohol on the central nervous system?

55. A crash after a cocaine high consists of a long period of _____.

56. What health problems are associated with adolescents addicted to narcotic drugs?

57. Why is it important that nurses who care for adolescents know whether the adolescents use drugs compulsively?

58. **T   F**   Depression is common in adolescents who commit suicide.

59. Differentiate between suicidal ideation and parasuicide.

60. Nursing care of the suicidal adolescent includes the following:
    a.

    b.

    c.

APPLYING CRITICAL THINKING TO THE NURSING PRACTICE

A. Spend a day in a gynecology clinic to oversee the diseases and disorders affecting the female reproductive system. Answer the following questions and include specific examples to illustrate these concepts.
   1. Besides pregnancy, what could lead to secondary amenorrhea?

   2. The nursing responsibilities in relation to sexually transmitted infections are all-encompassing. For each of the following nursing goals, identify one appropriate intervention to accomplish this goal.
      a. Informing the patient of the condition

Chapter **16   Health Problems of School-Age Children and Adolescents**

b. Primary prevention of sexually transmitted infections (STIs)

c. Tertiary prevention through treatment

B. Answer the following questions about obesity in adolescence.
1. Why is obesity considered a major problem of adolescence?

2. An obese adolescent tells the nurse that her obesity is a result of her low metabolism. What is the nurse's best response to this statement?

3. Formulate five nursing diagnoses that could apply to the obese adolescent.
a.

b.

c.

d.

e.

C. Answer the following questions related to eating disorders.
1. What lifestyle factor appears to be common to the initiation of both anorexia nervosa and bulimia nervosa?

2. What role does society have in the increased incidence of anorexia and bulimia?

D. Becky is a 16-year-old girl admitted to the adolescent unit after ingesting seven of her mother's pain pills with an unknown quantity of alcohol. After the drugs have been removed from her system and she has stabilized, Becky tells the nurse that she is so stressed out by her parents' recent divorce that she wishes she were dead.

1. In assessing Becky's family status, what factors might the nurse discover?

2. What are the most important nursing interventions for preventing further suicide attempts?

17 Quality of Life for Children Living with Chronic or Complex Diseases

Chapter 17 introduces nursing considerations essential to the care of the child with a chronic illness, disability, or terminal illness. At the completion of this chapter, the student will understand the impact that a diagnosis of a chronic illness or disability has on both the child and family and be able to develop appropriate nursing interventions to assist each family member in adjusting and developing to his or her fullest potential, despite the disability. The student will also be prepared to provide family-centered end-of-life care.

REVIEW OF ESSENTIAL CONCEPTS

Perspectives on the Care of Children with Special Needs

1. Attention is focused on what three aspects to emphasize the child's abilities and strengths rather than disabilities?
   a.

   b.

   c.

2. Part of family-centered care is having effective _____ and _____ between parents and nurses to form trusting and effective partnerships.

3. Clinicians need to know that siblings of children with chronic illnesses are at risk for _____.

4. List four factors that have been found to influence parent dissatisfaction with the communication between themselves and the health care system.
   a.

   b.

   c.

   d.

5. What is an important first step in formulating a plan for families of other cultural backgrounds?

The Family of the Child with a Chronic or Complex Condition

6. Identify two critical times for parents of children with a chronic or complex condition.

   a.

   b.

7. List the adaptive tasks of parents who have children with chronic conditions.

   a.

   b.

   c.

   d.

   e.

   f.

   g.

   h.

8. Identify two ways parents can promote healthy sibling relationships for children with special needs.

   a.

   b.

9. Define *empowerment*.

10. Identify three types of denial in family members that may be exhibited at the time a child is diagnosed with a chronic illness or disability.

   a.

   b.

   c.

11. Name four common responses of parents that manifest during the adjustment stage.

   a.

   b.

   c.

   d.

12. Match the four types of parental reaction during the period of adjustment to the appropriate behavior

   a. _____ Overprotection

   b. _____ Rejection

   c. _____ Denial

   d. _____ Gradual acceptance

   1. Parents place necessary and realistic restrictions on the child
   2. Parents act as if the disorder does not exist
   3. Parents detach themselves emotionally from the child
   4. Parents avoid discipline and cater to every desire of the child

13. Identify six variables that influence the resolution of a crisis in families.

   a.

   b.

   c.

   d.

   e.

   f.

14. **T   F**   The level of adjustment is significantly influenced by the level of technology dependence of the child.

126

15. **T   F**   The child's reaction to chronic illness depends on his or her temperament and coping mechanisms.

16. **T   F**   The impact of a chronic illness or disability on a child is influenced by the age of onset.

17. Identify the two maladaptive coping patterns found in children with special needs that are associated with poorer adaptation.
    a.

    b.

18. How can having a sense of hope help adolescent children with special needs?

19. **T   F**   Children with *less* severe disorders often cope better than those with *more* severe conditions.

Nursing Care of the Family and Child with a Chronic or Complex Condition

20. Why must assessment of the family and child with special needs be a continuous process?

21. Which question can the nurse ask to evaluate the parents' coping mechanism?
    a. Do you live near a tertiary medical center?
    b. Is your child's personality easy, difficult, or in-between?
    c. Does the child have siblings?
    d. Have you ever worked in the medical field?

22. What is the best way for the nurse to end the informing conference with the family of a child with special needs?

23. Identify a way in which the nurse can reduce anxiety in children with special needs?

24. What is an extension of revealing the diagnosis?

25. What can be done to promote normal development in the child with a chronic or complex condition?

26. One of the most difficult adjustments of parents with a special-needs child is the ability to set

    _____ for the child.

27. Because adolescence is a time of enormous physical and emotional changes, it is important for the nurse to make a

    distinction between _____ that are related to the child's complex condition and those that
    are a result of normal body development.

Perspectives on the Care of Children at the End of Life

28. List three factors that affect the causes of death that nurses are likely to encounter in children.
    a.

    b.

    c.

29. What are the goals for hospice care for children?

30. Differentiate between assisted suicide and euthanasia.

Nursing Care of the Child and Family at the End of Life

31. List some of the fears usually experienced by the terminally ill child and his or her family.
    a.

    b.

    c.

32. In the final hours of life, the dying patient's respiration may become labored, with deep breaths and long periods of apnea; this is referred to as _____ respirations. What should the nurse reassure families about when the dying patient has labored respirations?

33. **T** **F** After the child's death, the family should be allowed to remain with the body and hold or rock the child if they desire.

34. **T** **F** Grief is an event that that is orderly and predictable.

35. **T** **F** Complicated grief reactions can occur more than 1 year after the child's death.

36. Which nursing care intervention can support a grieving family?
    a. Provide rationalizations for the child's death, such as "Your child isn't suffering anymore"
    b. Offer consolidation such as "You are still young enough to have another baby"
    c. Ignore feelings of guilt or anger with the parents
    d. Sit quietly with the family

37. List four strategies that can assist nurses in maintaining their ability to work effectively.
    a.

    b.

    c.

    d.

APPLYING CRITICAL THINKING TO THE NURSING PRACTICE

A. The hospice nurse is caring for a dying child and her family. The nurse must understand the following in order to give the family and child the best patient care.
   1. What kind of information to dying children is needed from a nurse?

   2. When is it acceptable to withhold or withdraw treatments that cause pain and suffering and instead provide interventions that promote comfort?

B. Answer the following questions related to the care of a child with a chronic health problem in the home.
   1. What does home care represent?

Chapter **17** **Quality of Life for Children Living with Chronic or Complex Diseases**

2. What three goals does home care seek to achieve?
   a.

   b.

   c.

C. Interview the parents of a child with a disability to determine the family's adjustment. Answer the following questions and include specific responses to illustrate these concepts.
   1. Identify three areas that the nurse should assess when determining the adequacy of a family's support systems.
      a.

      b.

      c.

   2. Why is it necessary for the nurse to assess the family's specific perceptions concerning the illness or disability?

   3. Briefly describe the following behaviors that might be observed in a child who has coped with a disability.
      a. Competence and optimism
      b. Feeling different and withdraws
      c. Complies with treatment
      d. Seeks support
   4. What are the basic nursing goals for families and children with special needs?
      a.

      b.

      c.

      d.

      e.

      f.

D. Interview children in various age groups to determine their perceptions of death. Answer the following questions and include specific responses to illustrate these concepts.
   1. How do children between the ages of 3 and 5 years of age view death?

   2. If a preschooler becomes seriously ill, how is he or she likely to perceive the illness?

   3. Between what years of age do most children have an adult concept of death?

   4. Identify at least five nursing interventions that could be used when caring for a terminally ill adolescent in the hospital.
      a.

      b.

      c.

      d.

      e.

E. A child is dying in a hospital. The child's family has many questions and concerns related to the child's impending death. Answer the following questions related to this situation.
   1. How can the nurse assist the parents of a child who is dying in the hospital after an accident, trauma, or acute illness?
      a.

      b.

      c.

   2. How can the nurse control the environment to provide family-centered end-of-life care to this child and family?
      a.

      b.

Chapter **17** **Quality of Life for Children Living with Chronic or Complex Diseases**

c.

d.

3. What is the nurse's role in providing family-centered care after the child's death?

4. Describe the nurse's role in discussing organ or tissue donation with the family of a terminally ill child.

5. A family might have concerns about whether they can have an open-casket burial if they decide to donate their child's organs or tissue. What is the best response a nurse can give to this question?

18 Impact of Cognitive or Sensory Impairment on the Child and Family

Chapter 18 introduces nursing considerations essential to the care of the child with a cognitive impairment or a sensory or communication disorder. Cognitive or sensory impairments can pose a threat to the child's potential development; therefore it is important for students to understand specific issues related to the care of children with these types of disorders. This knowledge will enable the student to develop nursing strategies that will promote optimum achievement of the child's potential.

REVIEW OF ESSENTIAL CONCEPTS

Cognitive Impairment

1. Intellectual disability in children, as defined by the American Association on Intellectual and Developmental Disabilities, consists of which three components?
   a. Intellectual functioning, functional strengths and weaknesses, and age older than 18 years at time of diagnosis
   b. Intellectual functioning, physical strengths and weaknesses, and age younger than 18 years at time of diagnosis
   c. Intellectual functioning, functional strengths and weaknesses, and age younger than 18 years at time of diagnosis
   d. Intellectual functioning, physical strengths and weaknesses, and age older than 18 years at time of diagnosis

2. Which of the following is a new recommendation by the American Psychiatric Association's *Diagnostic and Statistical Manual of Mental Disorders*, Fifth Edition (DSM-5), for cognitive impairment?
   a. Rely on measures of social responsibility instead of intelligence quotient (IQ).
   b. Rely on IQ as the primary factor for determining cognitive impairment.
   c. Rely on measures of social independence instead of IQ.
   d. Move away from exclusively relying on IQ testing toward using additional measures of adaptive functioning.

3. What are three early signs of cognitive impairment in children?
   a.

   b.

   c.

4. _____ can be described as any significant lag or delay in a child's physical, cognitive, behavioral, emotional, or social development when compared with developmental norms.

5. Which of the following are most recognized as being the primary causes of cognitive impairment?
   a. Environmental, genetic, and infectious
   b. Genetic, biochemical, and infectious
   c. Genetic, organic, and social
   d. Environmental, organic, and social

6. A child is diagnosed with a cognitive impairment. The nurse notes the history and understands that which of the following is most consistent with the potential cause of cognitive impairment in this child?
   a. Postmaturity
   b. Maternal diabetes
   c. Maternal age
   d. Congenital rubella

7. The nurse caring for a child with cognitive impairment understands that which of the following nursing interventions is most effective when trying to communicate with the child?
   a. A variety of stimuli should be offered at the same time.
   b. Verbal explanation is preferred to demonstration.
   c. Demonstration is preferred to verbal explanation.
   d. Learning should be directed toward understanding principals.

8. When a nurse is teaching self-help skills to the family of a child with cognitive deficits, what two factors are important to assess before giving the instruction?
   a.

   b.

9. A nurse is assessing a child and notes that he has long, wide, protruding ears; a long, narrow face with prominent jaw; strabismus; hypotonia; and moderate cognitive impairment. What condition is characterized by these clinical manifestations?
   a. Down syndrome
   b. Fragile X syndrome
   c. Lupus
   d. Fetal alcohol syndrome

10. Which supplement is associated with the prevention of neural tube defects in newborns if taken during pregnancy?
    a. Vitamin K
    b. Folic acid
    c. Vitamin D
    d. Iron

11. What is the most common chromosomal abnormality of a generalized syndrome?
    a. Down syndrome
    b. Neural tube defects
    c. Cerebral palsy
    d. Fragile X syndrome

12. **T F** The majority (about 80%) of infants with Down syndrome are born to women younger than 35 years?

13. The nurse cares for a newborn baby and upon assessment notes the following: separated sagittal suture, brachycephaly, flat occiput, inner epicanthal folds, depressed nasal bridge, protruding tongue, short and broad neck. What do these clinical manifestations suggest?
    a. Fragile X syndrome
    b. Down syndrome
    c. Neural tube defect
    d. Meningitis

Sensory Impairment

14. Define the following terms.
    a. Hearing impaired

    b. Deaf

    c. Hard-of-hearing

15. Differentiate between conductive and sensorineural hearing loss.

16. When the conductive loss is permanent, hearing can be improved with the use of a _____.

17. What is used for treating sensorineural hearing loss?
    a. Cochlear implant
    b. Hearing aid
    c. Antibiotic therapy
    d. Tympanostomy tubes

18. Differentiate among the following terms used to describe receptive-expressive disorders caused by an organic central auditory defect.
    a. Aphasia
    b. Agnosia
    c. Dysacusis

19. What is the common treatment of conductive hearing loss?
    a. Antibiotic treatment
    b. Hearing aid
    c. Cochlear implant
    d. No treatment is indicated

20. Which of the following interventions is appropriate for reducing whistling noise from a hearing aid?
    a. Pushing the hearing aid further inside the canal.
    b. Increasing the volume on the hearing aid.
    c. Cleaning out the ear canal.
    d. Removing the aid.

21. Match the type of refractive error with its defining characteristics. (Answers may be used more than once.)

    a. _____ Myopia
    b. _____ Hyperopia
    c. _____ Anisometropia
    d. _____ Astigmatism

    1. Also referred to as farsightedness
    2. Also referred to as nearsightedness
    3. Refers to unequal curvatures in the cornea or lens so that light rays are bent in different directions, producing a blurred image
    4. Refers to the ability to see objects clearly at close range but not at a distance
    5. Refers to a difference of refractive strength in each eye
    6. Corrected with special lenses that compensate for refractive errors
    7. Refers to the ability to see objects clearly at a distance
    8. Biconcave lenses used in the correction of defect
    9. Treated with corrective lenses to improve vision in each eye so that the eyes work as a unit
    10. Convex lenses used in the correction of defect

22. When should a child be referred for a hearing evaluation?
    a. Absence of well-formed syllables by 8 months of age
    b. Absence of well-formed syllables by 9 months of age
    c. Absence of well-formed syllables by 10 months of age
    d. Absence of well-formed syllables by 11 months of age

23. Because the most common cause of impaired hearing in children is chronic otitis media, which of the following is a primary nursing role?
    a. Proper administration of antibiotics
    b. Annual hearing screens for children
    c. Prevention of hearing loss
    d. Routine immunizations

Chapter **18** **Impact of Cognitive or Sensory Impairment on the Child and Family**

24. What are some clues nurses can teach parents to determine whether infants are visually responding to them?

25. How do children who are both deaf and blind learn to communicate?

26. Describe the effects that auditory and visual impairment have on a child's development?

27. A nurse is caring for an infant and observes a whitish glow in the child's left pupil. What should the nurse do next?
    a. Report the finding to the physician because it could indicate glaucoma.
    b. Report the finding to the physician because it could indicate cataracts.
    c. Report the finding to the physician because it could indicate retinoblastoma.
    d. Simply document the finding because it is commonly observed in infants.

28. Describe typical characteristics of autism.

29. **T   F**   Autism appears to be caused by the measles-mumps-rubella (MMR) and thimerosal-containing vaccines.

APPLYING CRITICAL THINKING TO THE NURSING PRACTICE

A. A nursing student spends a day in a school with children of various cognitive impairments. Answer the following questions.
   1. What are some common early behavioral signs of a cognitive impairment in children?

   2. List at least two clinical manifestations of Down syndrome under each body system.
      a. Head and eyes

      b. Nose and ears

      c. Mouth and neck

      d. Chest and heart

e. Abdomen and genitalia

f. Hands and feet

g. Musculoskeletal system and skin

h. Other

3. A newly delivered infant is diagnosed with Down syndrome. What is the nurse's role in provided family-centered care to the child and his or her parents?
   a.

   b.

   c.

   d.

B. The nursing student observes testing, evaluation, and treatment modalities for a child with a visual impairment in a vision clinic. Answer the following questions and include specific examples to illustrate these concepts.
   1. Identify the various causes of visual impairment.

   2. For each of the following nursing goals, list at least three nursing interventions that would be used when caring for a child with a visual impairment and his or her family.
      a. Prevention of vision loss in infancy

      b. Detection of vision loss in childhood

   3. Nursing care related to caring for a blind child must include interventions aimed at teaching the child and family how to promote the child's independence in navigational skills. What are the two main techniques that promote this in blind children?
      a.

      b.

4. When the nurse is counseling the parents of an infant who is blind, what interventions would accomplish the goal "Promote parent-child attachment"?

   a.

   b.

C. Tom, age 2 years, is admitted for treatment of retinoblastoma. How can the nurse prepare Tom's parents for his postoperative appearance after enucleation of his affected eye?

D. Answer the following questions concerning the care for a child with autism spectrum disorders.
   1. What is known about the intellectual capacity of most autistic children?

   2. What assessment data are critical to implementing appropriate interventions and family involvement when caring for autistic children?

   3. Which children diagnosed with autism spectrum disorders have the most favorable prognosis?

19 Family-Centered Care of the Child During Illness and Hospitalization

Chapter 19 provides an overview of how children of various ages react to illness, pain, and hospitalization. After completing this chapter, the student will understand the different ways in which children and families react to the stress of illness, pain, and hospitalization. This chapter prepares the student to provide family-centered care of the child during illness and hospitalization.

REVIEW OF ESSENTIAL CONCEPTS

Stressors of Hospitalization and Children's Reactions

1. Which of the following is a manifestation of separation anxiety in infants?
   a. Biting strangers
   b. Forcing parents to stay
   c. Avoids and rejects contact with strangers
   d. Cries when parents enter room

2. A nurse is caring for a child who has been hospitalized for 12 days. The nurse notes that the child has become increasingly self-centered and is attaching primary importance to material objects. The nurse recognizes this as the

   _____ stage of separation anxiety.
   a. protest
   b. despair
   c. detachment
   d. acceptance

3. From middle infancy through preschool years, _____ is the major stressor related to hospitalization.

4. Identify some physiologic responses to stress in children.

5. **T F** Preschoolers are less secure interpersonally than toddlers, and therefore they cannot tolerate brief periods of separation from their parents.

6. Lack of _____ increases the perception of threat and can affect children's coping skills.
   a. sensory stimulation
   b. peer socialization
   c. rituals
   d. control

7. The needs of children vary with age. Match each of the following responses to a loss of control with the age group that the response exemplifies. (Answers can be used more than once.)

a. _____ They strive for autonomy and react with negativism to any physical restriction.

b. _____ Explanations are understood only in terms of real events.

c. _____ Their initial reaction to dependency is negativism and aggression.

d. _____ They respond with depression, hostility, and frustration to physical restrictions.

e. _____ They often voluntarily isolate themselves from age-mates until they can compete on an equal basis.

1. Toddlers
2. Preschoolers
3. School-age children
4. Adolescents

8. Which of the following situations is the most likely to result in anxiety in a hospitalized child?
   a. A child who lives in an urban area being admitted to the hospital
   b. A child who lives in a rural area being admitted to the hospital
   c. A child who is active and strong willed being admitted to the hospital
   d. A child who receives frequent family visits after being admitted to the hospital

9. List the individual risk factors that increase a child's vulnerability to the stresses of hospitalization.
   a.

   b.

   c.

   d.

   e.

   f.

10. **T   F**   Without special attention devoted to meeting the child's psychosocial and developmental needs in the hospital environment, the detrimental consequences of prolonged hospitalization may be severe.

Stressors and Reactions of the Family of the Child Who Is Hospitalized

11. Identify some common themes concerning stressors and reactions of the family of the child who is hospitalized.

12. Which of the following factors specific to the hospital experience have been found to have a negative effect on the siblings of a child who is hospitalized?
    a. Being older and experiencing few changes
    b. Being cared for outside the home by care providers who are not relatives
    c. Receiving detailed information about their ill brother or sister
    d. Perceiving that their parents treat them the same way they treated them before their sibling's hospitalization

140

Nursing Care of the Child Who Is Hospitalized

13. The rationale for preparing children for the hospital experience and related procedures is based on the principle that

    fear of the _____ exceeds fear of the _____.

14. The nurse is caring for a hospitalized child. The nurse notes that the child seems detached from his parents. Which of the following interventions can the nurse employ to help the child from detaching from his parents?
    a. Avoiding talking about the child's parents
    b. Educating the parents that this is normal and to be expected
    c. Stressing the importance of social visits from friends
    d. Frequently talking positively about the child's parents

15. A primary nursing goal when a child is hospitalized (particularly children 5 years old or younger) is to prevent

    negative effects from _____.

16. Describe family-centered care as a philosophy of care.

17. What four actions can the nurse take to minimize feelings of loss of control?
    a.

    b.

    c.

    d.

18. The dependent role of the hospitalized patient imposes tremendous feelings of loss on older children. Which of the following interventions should the nurse implement to help promote individuality in the hospitalized child?
    a. Encourage the child to stay in bed and watch his or her favorite TV show.
    b. Encourage the child to make decisions about his or her daily routine.
    c. Encourage the child to use the time in the hospital to catch up on schoolwork.
    d. Encourage the child to conform to the routines set in the hospital.

19. Because of toddlers' and preschool children's poorly defined body boundaries, the use of _____ is helpful after drawing blood.
    a. restraints
    b. a tourniquet
    c. bandages
    d. pictures

20. What is an important nursing intervention for children who fear mutilation of body parts?

Chapter **19** Family-Centered Care of the Child During Illness and Hospitalization

21. Why is it important for nurses to be keenly aware of the medical terminology and vocabulary that they use every day when working with children?

22. List two ways the nurse can alter the perception of a child who is upset about his or her illness.
    a.

    b.

23. **T F**   A primary goal of nursing care for the child who is hospitalized is to minimize threats to the child's development.

24. Identify three nursing interventions that can be used to help children resume school activities while hospitalized.
    a.

    b.

    c.

25. _____ is one of the most important aspects of a child's life and one of the most effective tools for managing stress.
    a. Socialization
    b. Routines
    c. Watching TV
    d. Play

26. What are three of the various functions of play in the hospital?
    a.

    b.

    c.

27. A nurse is caring for a 10-year-old child who has been hospitalized for 16 days. Which of the following is the best nursing intervention for a child who has been hospitalized for a length of time and whose parents are unable to visit frequently?
    a. Have the parents bring a box with several small, inexpensive, brightly wrapped items with a different day of the week printed on the outside of each package.
    b. Have the parents hire a nanny who can sit in the hospital room with the child.
    c. Have the parents send a calendar with a count down to the next day they will be able to visit.
    d. Have the parents call the hospital daily with an update on the child's progress.

28. Match each type of play with its description or purpose.

a. _____ Offers the best opportunity for emotional expression, including the release of anger

b. _____ A psychologic technique reserved for use by trained therapists as an interpretative method

c. _____ A nondirective method for helping children deal with their concerns and fears

d. _____ Allows children to reenact frightening or puzzling hospital experiences

1. Play therapy
2. Therapeutic play
3. Dramatic play
4. Expressive activities

29. Identify two potential benefits of hospitalization to the child or family?

a.

b.

Nursing Care of the Family

30. The nurse understands that the preparation for discharge and home care begins
    a. when the physician writes the discharge order.
    b. two days before discharge.
    c. upon admission to the hospital.
    d. three days before discharge.

Care of the Child and Family in Special Hospital Situations

31. Identify the three benefits of ambulatory care.
    a.

    b.

    c.

32. When a child is placed in isolation, what is the best approach the nurse can take in preparing the young child to feel in control?

33. **T   F**   When parents first visit the child in the intensive care unit, the nurse should encourage them to sit with their child, while also instructing them about how their child will appear while hospitalized in the intensive care environment.

143

A. Paul, age 1 year, is admitted to the pediatric unit with a diagnosis of pneumonia. When his mother leaves the room, he screams and cries. As the nurse approaches Paul, he screams louder and turns away.

1. The nurse assesses Paul's behavior and understands it is a characteristic of the _____ stage of separation.

2. Paul had complications related to pneumonia and has now been hospitalized for a month. The nurse notices that when his mother leaves the room now, he does not cry and seems to be withdrawn from all people much of the

   time. The nurse understands his behavior is now characteristic of the _____ stage of separation.

3. What nursing interventions are appropriate for both stages of separation?

B. Kristi, 2 years old, is admitted to the pediatric unit with a diagnosis of influenza. She has been in the unit for the past 4 days and is now refusing to eat, demanding a bottle, and asking her mother to feed her. She is demonstrating anxiety related to the loss of control of her environment.
1. What is Kristi demonstrating through her behaviors?

2. Identify at least three appropriate nursing interventions that will help Kristi feel a sense of control over her environment.
   a.

   b.

   c.

C. Robert, 4 years old, is admitted to the pediatric unit with a diagnosis of gastroenteritis.
1. List at least three nursing interventions to accomplish the nursing goal "Family will receive adequate support."
   a.

   b.

   c.

2. List at least three nursing interventions to accomplish the nursing goal "Child will experience positive relationships."

    a.

    b.

    c.

3. Identify play activities appropriate for Robert during hospitalization.

Chapter **19** **Family-Centered Care of the Child During Illness and Hospitalization**

20 Pediatric Variations of Nursing Interventions

Chapter 20 provides detailed information relating to specific nursing interventions employed in the nursing care of children. The chapter highlights the importance of providing family-centered nursing care with of the understanding that hospitalized children are separated from their usual environment and do not possess the capacity for abstract thinking and reasoning. After completing this chapter, the student will have the theoretical basis to safely implement nursing procedures with the pediatric population.

REVIEW OF ESSENTIAL CONCEPTS

General Concepts Related to Pediatric Procedures

1. Define informed consent.

2. What three conditions must be met for informed consent to be valid and legal?
   a.

   b.

   c.

3. **T   F**   When there are multiple procedures in one surgery, one universal consent is sufficient.

4. Which of the following situations is legally recognized as an emancipated minor?
   a. Live-in boyfriend
   b. Parents' divorce
   c. Pregnancy
   d. College student

5. List three interventions that can be used to reduce anxiety in children undergoing procedures.
   a.

   b.

   c.

6. **T   F**   Procedures should be performed in the child's room whenever possible.

7. The nurse is preparing a child for a medical procedure. The nurse notes that the child is highly active and distractible. What intervention is most appropriate for the nurse to implement?
   a. Shorter individualized preparation session
   b. Longer individualized preparation session
   c. Detailed individualized preparation session
   d. Slow-paced individualized preparation session

8. Why should hospital personnel encourage and allow children to express feelings?
   a. In order to discover if the child is experiencing fear
   b. Because behavior is children's primary means of communicating and coping
   c. In order to discover if the child is experiencing pain
   d. Because verbal communication is children's primary means of communicating and coping

9. One of the most effective interventions to encourage children to express their feelings is

   _____ play.

10. Match each common nursing procedure with the play activity that would best prepare the child for the experience.

    a. _____ Injections
    b. _____ Ambulation
    c. _____ Deep breathing
    d. _____ Increasing fluid intake

    1. Blowing bubbles
    2. Giving a toddler a push-pull toy
    3. Letting a child handle the syringe and vial, and giving give an "injection" to a doll
    4. Cutting gelatin into fun shapes

11. Clinical observations show that _____ decreases anxiety in children and reduces the need for heavy doses of preoperative sedation.
    a. antianxiety medications
    b. exercise
    c. parental presence
    d. visualization

12. When might preoperative medication be unnecessary?

13. A nurse is caring for a child after pediatric surgery. Which of the following is the most appropriate nursing intervention for this situation?
    a. To elicit the child to communicate frequently and provide comfort
    b. To assess the child's range of motion frequently and provide comfort
    c. To assess the child's bowel sounds frequently and provide comfort
    d. To assess the child's pain frequently and administer analgesics to provide comfort

14. A nurse is caring for a 2-year-old child who is about to undergo a painful procedure. Which of the following is the best intervention for the nurse to use to help the child cope?
    a. Distraction
    b. Soft music
    c. Warm compresses
    d. Guided imagery

15. A nurse is caring for a child postoperatively. The child has suddenly started experiencing elevated temperature, tachycardia, tachypnea, acidosis, muscle rigidity, and rhabdomyolysis. What do these symptoms characterize?
    a. Pneumothorax
    b. Malignant hyperthermia
    c. Malignant hypothermia
    d. Shock

16. What are three risk factors for skin breakdown in children?

    a.

    b.

    c.

17. A child is immobile after surgery. What does the nurse recognize to be the most common place for tissue breakdown to occur?
    a. Top of the feet
    b. Abdomen
    c. Bottom of the feet
    d. Thighs

18. Staging of pressure ulcers is used to classify the _____ of _____ that has occurred.

19. The nurse is caring for a child with ventilator-assisted pneumonia. The nurse recognizes that this condition is most often caused by
    a. a virus.
    b. closed suction systems.
    c. improper handwashing.
    d. bed position with the head of the bed elevated no higher than 15 degrees.

20. **T   F**   In a child who is dehydrated, it is helpful if the nurse forces fluids by awakening the child several times throughout the night to drink liquids.

21. In the following situations, when should the diet not be advanced?
    a. Increase in appetite
    b. Increase in bowel sounds
    c. Abdominal cramping or distention
    d. Weight gain

22. Elevated temperature is a common symptom of _____ in children.
    a. dehydration
    b. a virus
    c. illness
    d. pain

23. Match each term regarding body temperature with its definition.

    a. _____ Set point

    b. _____ Fever

    c. _____ Hyperthermia

    1. An elevation in set point such that body temperature is regulated at a higher level
    2. Occurs when body temperature exceeds set point; results from the body or external conditions creating more heat than the body can eliminate
    3. The temperature around which body temperature is regulated

24. Indicate whether each of the following statements regarding elevated temperature is true or false.
    a. **T F**   Environmental measures to reduce fever may be used if they are tolerated by the child and if they do not induce shivering.
    b. **T F**   Children's Motrin and Children's Advil are approved for fever reduction in children younger than 6 months of age.
    c. **T F**   The sponge bath should be restarted until the skin surface is warm or if the child feels chilled.
    d. **T F**   Antipyretics are of no value in hyperthermia.
    e. **T F**   Tepid water baths are not effective in hyperthermia.

Safety

25. Identify a special hazard for children associated with children in electronically controlled beds.

26. What can be used as a handy guide to determine whether a toy is a potential choking danger to a young child?
    a. A blanket
    b. A toilet paper roll
    c. A paper towel roll
    d. A pillow case

27. The nurse is caring for a postoperative child. Which of the following risk factors puts the child at high risk for falls?
    a. Short bed rest
    b. Normotensive
    c. Altered mental state
    d. Known effects of narcotics

28. Define the following terms related to infection control and provide an example of each.
    a. Standard precautions

    b. Transmission-based precautions

29. _____ is the most critical infection-control practice.

30. Define restraint.

31. **T F**   The nurse must have an order before applying a restraint to a patient.

32. What is the proper technique for holding an infant during a lumbar puncture to enlarge spaces between the vertebrae?

Collection of Specimens

33. The _____ reflex, in infants 4 to 6 months of age, causes crying, extension of the back, flexion of the extremities, and urination.
    a. Moro
    b. Babinski
    c. Perez
    d. tonic neck

34. Suprapubic aspiration is useful in clarifying the diagnosis of a suspected _____ in acutely ill infants.

35. **T   F**   When drawing a blood culture, the nurse should discard the first sample of blood and collect the second sample.

Administration of Medication

36. Why are newborns and premature infants particularly vulnerable to the harmful effects of drugs?

37. The most reliable method for determining children's dosages is to calculate the proportional amount of

    _____ to body weight.

38. What are the preferred sites for intramuscular injections in infants and small children?
    a.

    b.

39. **T   F**   The oral route is preferred for administering medications to children because of the ease of administration.

40. Identify a nursing intervention that can be used to help infants up to 11 months of age and children with neurologic impairments to swallow.

41. **T   F**   After administering a medication that has an opaque preparation like penicillin, the nurse should aspirate for blood. When aspirating, the nurse should look for blood at the *bottom* of the syringe, because blood may be drawn up through the column of penicillin.

Maintaining Fluid Balance

42. Identify two disadvantages of using the weighed-diaper method of fluid measurement?
    a.

    b.

43. _____ provides a rapid, safe, and lifesaving alternate route for the administration of fluids and medications until intravascular access can be attained, especially in children who are 6 years of age and or younger.

Procedures for Maintaining Respiratory Function

44. The organs most vulnerable to damage from excessive oxygenation (oxygen toxicity) are the

_____ and the _____.

45. Describe oxygen-induced carbon dioxide narcosis.

46. List the three advantages of oximetry over transcutaneous monitoring.
    a.

    b.

    c.

47. **T   F**   Bronchial drainage is more effective immediately after aerosol therapy.

48. When suctioning an infant with a tracheostomy, the nurse notes the vacuum pressure needs to remain between which of the following?
    a. 70 to 110 mm hg
    b. 40 to 80 mm hg
    c. 60 to 100 mm hg
    d. 40 to 60 mm hg

49. Air or gas delivered directly to the trachea must be _____.

50. A child with a tracheostomy may be unable to signal for help; therefore direct observation and use of

_____ and _____ monitors are essential.

Procedures Related to Alternative Feeding Techniques
51. What function does pH paper serve in nasogastric tube placement?

52. Children at high risk for regurgitation or aspiration, such as those children with gastroparesis, mechanical ventilation, or brain injuries, may require placement of a(n) _____ feeding tube.

53. Total parenteral nutrition (TPN) involves the intravenous (IV) infusion of highly concentrated solutions of a variety of elements, minerals, and other nutrients. List three elements that can be included in this mixture.

a.

b.

c.

Procedures Related to Elimination

54. Fleet enema is not recommended for children. What are the possible complications of this form of enema when used in children?

a.

b.

55. What is the most frequent cause of ostomies in infants?
a. Inflammatory bowel disease
b. Viral infections
c. Fevers
d. Necrotizing enterocolitis

APPLYING CRITICAL THINKING TO THE NURSING PRACTICE

A. Henry is admitted with a diagnosis of meningitis and a fever of 39.4° C (103° F).
1. How and when should the nurse evaluate whether the administration of an antipyretic has been effective?

2. What nursing interventions will help reduce Henry's fever?

3. During discharge teaching, what educational instructions should the nurse give to the parents regarding care of a child who has a fever?

B. Danny, age 3 months, is a patient on the pediatric unit. He is in elbow restraints after a cleft lip repair.
1. A nursing diagnosis is "risk of harm if sutures are removed, dislodged, or ruptured." What nursing interventions could be performed to ensure safety while the child is in restraints?

2. What safety measures must be taken to ensure that the restraints are properly secured?

C. Evan, age 6 months, is a patient on the pediatric unit. He is admitted to the unit in severe respiratory distress. He is placed in a mist tent in 35% oxygen.
  1. What interventions could the nurse implement to decrease Evan's fear of the mist tent?
    a.

    b.

    c.

  2. How should the nurse perform chest physiotherapy on Evan?

  3. How should the nurse evaluate whether the chest physiotherapy was successful in removing excess fluid?

D. The nurse is caring for a child with a tracheostomy.
  1. What complications should the nurse monitor in the child who has a tracheostomy?

  2. What is the focus of nursing care when caring for a child who has a tracheostomy?

  3. What should the nurse assess in the child to determine whether the lungs need to be suctioned?

  4. When suctioning the child's tracheostomy, the nurse should hyperventilate the child with 100% oxygen before and after suctioning. What is the underlying rationale for this action?

Chapter **20** **Pediatric Variations of Nursing Interventions**

21 The Child with Respiratory Dysfunction

Chapter 21 introduces nursing considerations essential to the care of the child experiencing respiratory dysfunction. Respiratory dysfunction is often more serious in young children. After completing this chapter, the student will be able to formulate nursing goals and identify nursing responsibilities to help the child and family effectively cope with the physical, emotional, and psychosocial stressors imposed by an alteration in respiratory function.

REVIEW OF ESSENTIAL CONCEPTS

Respiratory Infection

1. What accounts for the majority of acute illnesses in children?

2. What factors influence the etiology and course of respiratory infections in children?
   a.

   b.

   c.

   d.

3. Explain why anatomic size is a significant variable in respiratory tract infections of children.

4. Indicate whether each of the following statements is true or false.

   a. **T F**   Newborns (<28 days) may not develop a fever, even with severe infections.
   b. **T F**   The 6-month-old to 3-year-old may develop a high fever (39.5° to 40.5° C; 103° to 105° F) even with a mild respiratory illness.
   c. **T F**   Meningeal signs without infection of the meninges may be present in small children who have an abrupt onset of fever.
   d. **T F**   Vomiting is unlikely to occur with a respiratory tract infection.
   e. **T F**   A small child with a respiratory tract infection is unlikely to complain of abdominal pain.

5. What can a nurse instruct a family to do at home with a child who is experiencing mild respiratory symptoms, such as a stuffy nose caused by mucosal swelling?

6. What instructions can a nurse give a family on how to suction an infant who is going home but still has mucosal swelling?

Upper Respiratory Tract Infections

7. Differentiate between the clinical manifestations of nasopharyngitis in younger and older children. Match each item with the correct responses (more than one answer will apply to each).

   a. _____ Younger child

   b. _____ Older child

   1. Fever
   2. Irritability and poor feeding
   3. Dryness and irritation of the throat and nose
   4. Cough
   5. Decreased fluid intake
   6. Mouth breathing
   7. Vomiting or diarrhea
   8. Muscle aches

8. Are over-the-counter cold preparations such as pseudoephedrine appropriate for the treatment of the common cold in infants or toddlers? Why or why not?

9. Why are throat cultures often performed in children who present with acute pharyngitis?

10. What is the treatment for streptococcal throat infection?

11. Children with pharyngitis are considered infectious to others at the onset of symptoms and up to how many hours after initiation of antibiotic therapy? They should not return to school or daycare until they have been taking antibiotics for how long?

12. What filters and protects the respiratory and alimentary tracts from invasion by pathogenic organisms and plays a role in antibody formation?

13. What are the typical symptoms of tonsillitis?

14. List two instances in which a tonsillectomy is recommended.
    a.

    b.

15. What is a complication of a tonsillectomy and adenoidectomy signaled by frequent clearing of the throat or swallowing?

16. Why should children who have viral symptoms not receive aspirin?

17. Define the following terms.
    a. Otitis media

    b. Acute otitis media

    c. Otitis media with effusion

18. What does visual inspection of the tympanic membrane reveal in acute otitis media (AOM)?

19. Current literature indicates that waiting up to how many hours for spontaneous resolution is safe and appropriate management of AOM without severe signs and symptoms in healthy infants over 6 months?

20. When antimicrobial drug therapy is needed, what is the first drug of choice in the treatment of AOM?

21. What can be done to reduce the incidence of AOM in infants and children?

22. Which virus is the principal cause of infectious mononucleosis and is thought to be transmitted through saliva by direct intimate contact?

23. Identify eight early symptoms of mononucleosis.
    a.

    b.

    c.

    d.

    e.

    f.

    g.

    h.

24. Describe the "spot test" for diagnosing infectious mononucleosis.

25. What clinical manifestations of infectious mononucleosis require medical attention?

Croup Syndromes
26. What are the characteristics of croup symptoms?

27. Define *acute epiglottitis*.

28. What three clinical observations are predictive of epiglottitis?

a.

b.

c.

29. Describe the following areas of assessment characteristic of a child with epiglottitis.

a. Voice

b. Chest

c. Color

d. Throat

30. Why should the nurse not use a tongue depressor to examine the throat of a child with suspected epiglottitis?

31. What is the most common type of croup syndrome?

Infections of the Lower Airways

32. **T F** Bronchitis is frequently associated with upper respiratory infections and is usually self-limiting.

33. **T F** Severe respiratory syncytial virus (RSV) infections in the first year of life represent a significant risk factor for the development of asthma up to age 13.

34. Describe the pathophysiology of RSV.

35. **T F** Ribavirin should only be used for treatment of RSV in patients at high risk for mortality.

36. What precautions are employed with patients who have RSV?

37. The most useful classification of pneumonia is based on what?

38. Identify at least three organisms that cause pneumonia in school-age children.
    a.

    b.

    c.

39. What interventions can assist infants in handling secretions?

Other Infections of the Respiratory Tract

40. _____ is an acute respiratory infection caused by *Bordetella pertussis* that occurs primarily in children younger than 4 years of age who have not been immunized.

41. The causative organism in tuberculosis (TB) is _____.

42. In TB, the _____ is the usual portal of entry for the organism.

43. Medical management of TB in children consists of which six factors?
    a.

    b.

    c.

    d.

    e.

    f.

44. What type of precautions and room are required for children who are contagious and hospitalized with active TB disease?

45. The only certain means to prevent TB is to _____ with the tubercle bacillus.

46. The success of TB therapy depends on _____ with the drug regimen.

Pulmonary Dysfunction Caused by Noninfectious Irritants

47. **T   F**   Small children characteristically explore matter with their mouths and are prone to aspirate a foreign body.

48. What does laryngotracheal obstruction most commonly cause?
    a.

    b.

    c.

    d.

49. _____ is required for a definitive diagnosis of objects in the larynx and trachea.

50. What two lifesaving procedures should a nurse be able to implement to treat aspiration of a foreign body?
    a.

    b.

51. Identify which child is in severe respiratory distress.
    a. A child who can whisper for help, is mildly cyanotic, and is standing.
    b. A child who cannot speak, is mildly cyanotic, and is sitting in a chair.
    c. A child who cannot speak, is mildly cyanotic, and collapses.

52. **T   F**   Acute respiratory distress syndrome rarely occurs in children.

53. What are children more at risk for when they are exposed to (second-hand) passive tobacco smoke?

Long-Term Respiratory Dysfunction

54. List the reasons for the increase in morbidity and mortality rates related to asthma in the United States.
    a.

b.

c.

d.

e.

55. Indicate whether each of the following statements is true or false.
   a. **T F** Boys are affected by asthma more frequently than girls until adolescence.
   b. **T F** Children may experience asthma symptoms that range from acute episodes of shortness of breath, wheezing, and cough followed by a quiet period, to a relatively continuous pattern of chronic symptoms that fluctuate in severity.

56. Which are effective methods to evaluate the presence of lung disease in a child with a history of asthma? (Select all that apply.)
   a. Pulmonary function tests in a 4-year-old child
   b. Pulmonary function tests in a 6-year-old child
   c. Peak expiratory flow meter readings on a 10-year-old child who uses the device only during asthmatic episodes
   d. Peak expiratory flow meter readings on an 8-year-old child who regularly uses the device

57. What is the goal of drug therapy in asthma management for each of the two general classes?
   a. Long-term control medications

   b. Quick-relief medications

58. What class of drugs are antiinflammatory drugs used to treat reversible airflow obstruction?

59. What are the major therapeutic agents for treatment of acute exacerbations and prevention of exercise-induced bronchospasm?

60. How can breathing exercises and physical training help a child with asthma?

61. Describe exercise-induced bronchospasm.

Chapter **21** **The Child with Respiratory Dysfunction**

62. Describe the recent changes in recommendations related to hyposensitization of children.

63. Define *status asthmaticus*.

64. What are the drugs of choice for treating status asthmaticus?

65. How can the nurse develop a partnership between the child with asthma, the family, and the health care team?
    a.

    b.

    c.

66. Identify 10 objective signs of bronchospasm in children.
    a.

    b.

    c.

    d.

    e.

    f.

    g.

    h.

i.

j.

67. What clinical features characterize cystic fibrosis (CF)?
   a.

   b.

   c.

   d.

68. The primary factor of cystic fibrosis, and the one responsible for many of its clinical manifestations, is

   _____, which is caused by the increased viscosity of mucous gland secretions.

69. What role does meconium ileus have in the manifestation of cystic fibrosis?

70. Describe the effects of thickened secretions on the gastrointestinal tract of the child with cystic fibrosis.

71. Describe the stools of the child with cystic fibrosis.

72. What is a common gastrointestinal complication associated with cystic fibrosis?

73. A unique diagnostic characteristic of the child with cystic fibrosis is an increased amount of _____

   and _____ in the sweat.

74. What management is used to prevent and treat pulmonary infections?

75. Pancreatic enzymes are administered to the child with cystic fibrosis. Answer the following questions regarding the guidelines for administering the enzymes.

   a. When are they administered?

   b. Upon what does the dosage depend?

   c. Why is the amount of enzyme adjusted?

76. Describe the suggested diet for children with cystic fibrosis.

77. What has allowed survival rates for CF patients to improve?

78. Identify common symptoms of obstructive sleep-disordered breathing.

   a.

   b.

   c.

   d.

   e.

79. A common treatment for sleep-disordered breathing in children is _____.

Respiratory Emergency

80. Describe the two types of respiratory insufficiency.

   a.

   b.

81. Differentiate between respiratory arrest and apnea.

82. What are the cardinal signs of respiratory failure?

83. Indicate whether each of the following statements is true or false.
   a. **T** **F** When a child's airway is obstructed, the nurse should attempt to remove the object by a blind finger sweep of the mouth.
   b. **T** **F** The victim of a motor vehicle accident should be placed in the recovery position if rescue breathing or cardiopulmonary resuscitation (CPR) is required.

APPLYING CRITICAL THINKING TO THE NURSING PRACTICE

A. Rick, age 12 months, comes to urgent care with a fever of 39.4° C (103° F), rhinitis, nasal congestion, irritability, and difficulty feeding. He is diagnosed with an acute upper respiratory tract infection.
   1. List two possible nursing diagnoses for Rick.
      a.

      b.

   2. Identify two nursing interventions that could help alleviate his nasal congestion.
      a.

      b.

B. Ally, a 1-year-old girl, comes into the pediatrician's office with complaints of ear pain, a low-grade fever of 37.2° C (99° F), irritability, rhinitis, cough, difficulty sleeping, and poor appetite over the past 3 days. On inspection, the physician notes a purulent, discolored effusion and a bulging, reddened, immobile tympanic membrane. She is diagnosed with acute otitis media (AOM).
   1. What does current literature suggest in treating AOM in a 1-year-old child?

   2. What signs of AOM would you teach her parents to look for that indicate a possible infection?

C. Jenna, age 16 years, is admitted to the adolescent unit with a severe sore throat, persistent fever, fatigue, and general malaise. A diagnosis of infectious mononucleosis is made.
   1. How is infectious mononucleosis diagnosed?

   2. Jenna asks the nurse how she got mononucleosis. What is the nurse's best response to this question?

165

3. How would the nurse prepare Jenna for the Monospot test?

4. What are the nursing goals in caring for Jenna?
   a.

   b.

D. Sandy, the mother of Billy, age 2, comes to the emergency department with a chief complaint that her son went to bed with a low-grade fever and woke up 4 hours later with a barky, brassy cough. The nurse notes Billy has inspiratory stridor and suprasternal retractions. On further examination, it is discovered that Billy has an inflamed mucosal lining of the larynx and trachea. He is now coughing loudly and has a hoarse voice. Sandy says he developed a runny nose 3 days ago.
   1. It is highly likely that Billy has what condition?

   2. At what point did Billy's symptoms of hypoxia become evident and why?

   3. What can this type of obstruction lead to?

   4. What is the most important nursing function in the care of children with acute laryngotracheobronchitis?

   5. What is the rationale for the use of high humidity with cool mist?

E. Darrin, a 3-month-old infant, is brought into the emergency department by his parents. He has had rhinorrhea and low-grade fever for the past 3 days. This evening, his mother noticed that his left eye was red and that he had begun coughing. Darrin has been refusing to nurse over the past 6 hours, appears slightly lethargic, and is extremely irritable. The enzyme-linked immunosorbent assay (ELISA) was positive for respiratory syncytial virus (RSV) antigen detection.
   1. The physician orders ribavirin. Why is the use of this drug controversial?

   2. What nursing intervention could the nurse implement to ensure that Darrin's nutritional needs are met?

F. Alice, a 6-year-old girl, came to the emergency department with acute respiratory distress. Her mother noted that she appeared "fine" but over the past 2 hours had begun to cough without production and seemed unable to catch her breath. There is a family history of asthma (her father) and hay fever (her mother).
   1. What are some typical signs and symptoms of an acute asthmatic attack?

2. As the attack progresses, what additional symptoms would the nurse expect to assess?

3. Alice will be treated with a beta2-adrenergic agent. Describe its intended effects and side effects.
   a. Intended effects

   b. Side effects

4. List the overall goals of asthma management that guide the nursing care plan for the child with asthma and the child's family.
   a.

   b.

   c.

   d.

   e.

5. What are some expected outcomes for the patient goal of "Child will not have chronic symptoms and recurrent exacerbations"?
   a.

   b.

   c.

6. What nonpharmacologic interventions could the nurse teach this family to prevent further asthma attacks?

22 The Child with Gastrointestinal Dysfunction

Chapter 22 presents disorders of the gastrointestinal tract that affect children. These disorders constitute one of the largest categories of illness in infancy and childhood. After completing this chapter, the student will be able to assess the child with alterations in gastrointestinal function, such as disorders that affect gastrointestinal motility and inflammatory and functional disorders. The chapter will help the student develop family-centered nursing plans and interventions to assist the child with gastrointestinal dysfunction.

REVIEW OF ESSENTIAL CONCEPTS

Gastrointestinal Dysfunction

1. List five factors that increase fluid requirements in children.
   a.

   b.

   c.

   d.

   e.

2. Why are infants and young children more vulnerable than older children and adults to alterations in fluid and electrolyte balance?

3. Infants lose a large amount of fluid at birth and maintain a larger amount of _____ than the adult until about 2 to 3 years of age. This contributes to greater and more rapid _____ during this age period.

4. Two-thirds of insensible water loss occurs through _____ and the remaining one-third is lost through the _____.

5. Why is the basal metabolic rate in infants and children higher than it is in adults?

6. Indicate whether each of the following statements are true or false.
   a. **T** **F** One of the best determinants of the extent of dehydration in infants and young children is body weight.
   b. **T** **F** Urine-specific gravity and serum urea nitrogen are reliable assessments for diagnosing dehydration in children.
   c. **T** **F** If a child with dehydration is not thirsty, oral rehydration should not be attempted.
   d. **T** **F** In patients with severe dehydration, the first priority is restoration of circulation with extracellular fluid volume to treat or prevent shock.

Disorders of Motility

7. Diarrheal disturbances involve various areas of the gastrointestinal system. Match the anatomic area with the correct term.

   a. _____ Stomach and intestines

   b. _____ Colon

   c. _____ Small intestine

   d. _____ Colon and intestines

   1. Enterocolitis
   2. Colitis
   3. Enteritis
   4. Gastroenteritis

8. What causes acute infectious diarrhea (infectious gastroenteritis)?

9. Malabsorption syndromes, inflammatory bowel disease, immunodeficiency, food allergy, or lactose intolerance causes what type of diarrhea?

10. Which of the following is a common clinical manifestation of diarrhea?
    a. Shock
    b. Overhydration
    c. Metabolic alkalosis
    d. Dehydration

11. _____ is the most important cause of serious gastroenteritis with 28% of all cases causing fatality.

12. Watery, explosive stools suggest _____; foul-smelling, greasy, bulky stools suggest

    _____.

13. Identify four major goals in the management of acute diarrhea.
    a.

    b.

    c.

    d.

14. List the four elements of essential education related to oral rehydration therapy for parents of children with diarrhea.

a.

b.

c.

d.

15. The best intervention for diarrhea in infants and children is _____.

16. **T   F**   *Constipation* is defined as the frequency of bowel movements.

17. Constipation in infancy is often related to _____, while _____ is the most common cause of constipation in early childhood.

18. List the three goals for the management of chronic constipation

a.

b.

c.

19. _____ is the absence of ganglion cells in the affected bowel, resulting in a lack of the enteric nervous system stimulation.

20. After the pull-through procedure for treatment of Hirschsprung disease _____ and _____ may occur and require further therapy.

21. _____ is a well-defined, complex, coordinated process that is under central nervous system control and is often accompanied by nausea and retching.

22. What are the goals in the management of vomiting?

23. Define *gastroesophageal reflux* (GER).

24. When does GER become a disease?

Recurrent and Functional Abdominal Pain

25. Describe the characteristics of recurrent abdominal pain.

Inflammatory Disorders

26. Identify the clinical manifestations of appendicitis.

a.

b.

c.

d.

e.

f.

g.

h.

i.

j.

k.

l.

27. What is the McBurney point?

28. Identify the symptomatic complications of Meckel diverticulum.
    a.

    b.

    c.

29. How is Meckel diverticulum treated?

30. Which has a better prognosis, Crohn disease or ulcerative colitis?

31. Children with _____ are usually seen with diarrhea, rectal bleeding, and mild growth restriction.

32. Children with _____ are usually seen with severe anorexia and weight loss.

33. A(n) _____ ulcer involves the mucosa of the stomach; a(n) _____ ulcer involves the pylorus or duodenum.

Hepatic Disorders

34. Hepatitis _____ virus has significantly declined since the introduction of a vaccine in 1995.

    It is spread via the _____ route.

35. Identify three possible routes of transmission of hepatitis B virus.
    a.

    b.

    c.

36. What type of hepatitis is the most common cause of chronic liver disease?

37. What is a diagnosis of hepatitis based on?
   a.

   b.

   c.

38. What are the most effective measures in the prevention and control of viral hepatitis?

39. List four factors that can cause severe liver damage in children.
   a.

   b.

   c.

   d.

40. What are the two main goals of therapeutic management of cirrhosis?
   a.

   b.

Structural Defects

41. **T   F**   Cleft palate is more common than cleft lip and palate.

42. **T   F**   Exposure to teratogens such as alcohol and cigarettes are associated with higher rates of oral clefting.

43. _____ is the most immediate nursing problem in the care of the newborn with cleft lip and palate deformities.

44. Management of cleft lip and cleft palate is directed toward what three factors?

    a.

    b.

    c.

45. What anomalies are associated with tracheal or esophageal atresia?

    a.

    b.

    c.

46. Differentiate between an incarcerated and strangulated hernia.

Obstructive Disorders

47. Obstruction in the gastrointestinal tract that occurs when the passage of nutrients and secretions is impeded by impaired motility is called a(n) _____.

48. Pyloric stenosis is characterized by _____ vomiting.

49. How does intussusception occur?

50. What is the peak range of age of intussusception?

51. **T   F**   Intussusception is more common in females than in males.

52. What sign indicates that the intussusception has reduced itself?

Malabsorption Syndromes

53. _____ is characterized by chronic diarrhea and malabsorption of nutrients.

54. List the clinical manifestations of celiac disease.
    a.

    b.

    c.

    d.

    e.

    f.

    g.

    h.

    i.

    j.

55. _____ can occur in celiac disease and is characterized by acute, severe episodes of profuse, watery diarrhea and vomiting.

56. The main nursing consideration in celiac disease is helping the child adhere to _____.

A. Kevin, age 3 years, is admitted to the hospital unit with a diagnosis of dehydration and acute diarrhea related to rotavirus infection.

   1. What is the priority nursing diagnosis?

   2. The nurse conducting the initial assessment on Kevin should note the following assessment findings that suggest dehydration.

      a.

      b.

      c.

      d.

      e.

      f.

      g.

      h.

   3. How much oral rehydration solution should be given to Kevin?

   4. What nursing intervention is essential to determine whether renal blood flow is sufficient to permit the addition of potassium to the intravenous fluids?

   5. How should the nurse instruct Kevin's parents with regard to diaper changing and the disposal of diapers to prevent the spread of the virus?

B. Bailey, a 4-month-old infant, is brought into the pediatric clinic for evaluation. Her mother reports that she spits up small amounts of formula after each feeding and fusses and cries after spitting up. Bailey has difficulty sleeping at night because she is irritable after feedings. The physician diagnosed her with gastroesophageal reflux (GER). Right now the treatment of choice is symptom management, because Bailey is gaining weight and thriving.

   1. Bailey's mother wants to know why there is nothing more they can do for Bailey. What is the best response by the nurse?

   2. What three suggestions could the nurse offer Bailey's mother that might help alleviate some of Bailey's discomfort?

     a.

     b.

     c.

   3. Bailey's mom wants to know if she should continue to breastfeed. What recommendations can you offer her regarding breastfeeding for an infant with GER?

C. Allen, age 10 years, is admitted for treatment of appendicitis.

   1. What is the first classic symptom of appendicitis?

   2. Peritonitis is a possible risk associated with a ruptured appendix. What are some signs of peritonitis the nurse should be aware of?

   3. What are the expected outcomes of the nursing goal of "Child will not experience abdominal distention"?

D. The nurse is caring for a child with ulcerative colitis (UC).

   1. What symptoms should the nurse expect a child with UC to manifest?

   2. When is surgery indicated for UC?

3. What long-term complication is associated with UC and Crohn disease that requires routine surveillance 10 years after diagnosis?

E. Samuel, age 11 years, was recently diagnosed with hepatitis B.
   1. The nursing goals for Samuel's care depend on what three factors?
      a.

      b.

      c.

   2. What should the nurse encourage Samuel and his family to do to promote healing and rest?

F. The nurse is caring for a child who has hypertrophic pyloric stenosis.
   1. When does this condition usually develop?

   2. What are the presenting symptoms?

   3. What nursing interventions with regard to infant feedings are instituted soon after surgery?

G. Patricia, age 3 years, is admitted with a diagnosis of celiac disease.
   1. A gluten-free diet usually produces dramatic clinical improvement within 2 weeks. How does the nurse teach Patricia's parents to adhere to this diet?

   2. What grains should be eliminated from Patricia's diet?

   3. What grains would be included in Patricia's diet?

   4. Which organization should the nurse refer the parents for help with a child diagnosed with celiac disease?

23 The Child with Cardiovascular Dysfunction

Chapter 23 introduces nursing considerations essential to the care of the child experiencing cardiovascular dysfunction. After completing this chapter, the student should have the information needed to provide family-centered care, develop appropriate nursing care plans, and implement appropriate interventions for the child with cardiovascular dysfunction.

REVIEW OF ESSENTIAL CONCEPTS

Cardiovascular Dysfunction

1. What is the first important step in assessing an infant or child for possible heart disease?
   a. Assessing for environmental factors
   b. Taking an accurate health history
   c. Taking the infant or child's vital signs
   d. Assessing for autoimmune responses

2. The nurse is caring for a newborn infant. Upon maternal history the nurse notes that the mother has a chronic health condition associated with heart disease in infants. Which of the following diseases is associated with heart disease in children?
   a. Diabetes and lupus
   b. Cystic fibrosis and lupus
   c. Multiple sclerosis and lupus
   d. Crohn disease and lupus

3. _____ involves the use of ultra high frequency sound waves and is one of the most frequently used tests for detecting cardiac dysfunction in children.

4. Which of the following is a complication that the nurse might assess after a cardiac catheterization?
   a. Hemorrhage at the entry site
   b. Rapidly rising blood pressure
   c. Hypostatic pneumonia
   d. Congestive heart failure

Congenital Heart Disease

5. The ductus arteriosus starts to close after birth in the presence of _____ in the blood and other factors.

6. Which risk factor contributes to an increased morbidity and mortality related to congenital heart disease?
   a. Postmaturity
   b. High birth weight
   c. Low birth weight
   d. Older age at time of surgery

7. The classification of acyanotic congenital heart defects is subdivided into the blood flow pattern groups of "increased pulmonary blood flow" and "obstruction to blood flow from ventricles." Match each of the following defects with the appropriate group.

a. _____ Atrial septal defect

b. _____ Pulmonic stenosis

c. _____ Aortic stenosis

d. _____ Ventricular septal defect

e. _____ Patent ductus arteriosus

f. _____ Atrioventricular canal defect

g. _____ Coarctation of the aorta

1. Increased pulmonary blood flow
2. Obstruction to blood flow from ventricles

8. Match the following definitions, clinical manifestations, or treatments with the appropriate congenital cardiac defect.

a. _____ An abnormal opening exists between the atria, allowing blood from the higher-pressure left atrium to flow to the lower-pressure right atrium.

b. _____ Patients are at risk for bacterial endocarditis and pulmonary vascular obstructive disease. Eisenmenger syndrome may develop.

c. _____ Incomplete fusion of endocardial cushions creates a large central atrioventricular valve, allowing blood to flow between all four chambers of the heart.

d. _____ This defect causes a characteristic machinelike murmur. Administration of indomethacin has proved successful in treating this.

e. _____ Patient has high blood pressure and bounding pulses in arms; weak or absent femoral pulses; and cool lower extremities with lower blood pressure.

f. _____ Narrowing occurs at the entrance to the pulmonary artery. Resistance to blood flow causes right ventricular hypertrophy and decreased pulmonary blood flow.

g. _____ The prominent anatomic consequence is hypertrophy of the left ventricular wall, leading to increased end diastolic pressure.

1. Atrial septal defect
2. Pulmonic stenosis
3. Patent ductus arteriosus
4. Ventricular septal defect
5. Atrioventricular canal defect
6. Coarctation of the aorta
7. Aortic stenosis

9. The classification of cyanotic congenital heart defects is subdivided into the blood flow pattern groups of "decreased pulmonary blood flow" and "mixed blood flow." Match each of the following defects with the appropriate group.

a. _____ Tetralogy of Fallot

b. _____ Tricuspid atresia

c. _____ Transposition of great arteries

d. _____ Total anomalous pulmonary venous return

e. _____ Truncus arteriosus

f. _____ Hypoplastic left heart syndrome

1. Decreased pulmonary blood flow
2. Mixed blood flow

10. Which of the following group of drugs is used to reduce the afterload on the heart and thus make it easier for the heart to pump?
    a. Digitalis glycosides
    b. Beta blockers
    c. Calcium channel blockers
    d. Angiotensin-converting enzyme inhibitors

11. Match the following conditions with the appropriate term.

    a. _____ The ventricle is unable to pump blood effectively into the pulmonary artery, resulting in increased pressure in the right atrium and systemic venous circulation.

    1. Left-sided failure
    2. Right-sided failure

    b. _____ The ventricle is unable to pump blood into the systemic circulation, resulting in increased pressure in the left atrium and pulmonary veins.

    c. _____ Systemic venous hypertension causes hepatosplenomegaly and occasionally edema.

    d. _____ The lungs become congested with blood, causing elevated pulmonary pressures and pulmonary edema.

12. Which of the following diagnostic evaluation tools can be used to assess for cardiomegaly and increased pulmonary blood flow?
    a. Clinical manifestations
    b. Chest radiography
    c. Echocardiogram
    d. Electrocardiogram

13. Coarctation of the aorta can cause _____ as a result of decreased cardiac output.
    a. bounding femoral pulses
    b. congestive heart failure
    c. hypotension
    d. pulmonary congestion

14. Which of the following procedures uses contrast material to illuminate heart structures and blood flow patterns?
    a. Cardiac catheterization
    b. Hemodynamics
    c. Angiography
    d. Doppler

15. Which of the following drugs blocks action of aldosterone, which promotes retention of sodium and excretion of potassium?
    a. Spironolactone (Aldactone)
    b. Chlorothiazide (Diuril)
    c. Furosemide (Lasix)
    d. ACE inhibitors

16. Identify three common signs of digoxin toxicity in children.
    a.

    b.

    c.

Chapter **23** **The Child with Cardiovascular Dysfunction**

17. ACE inhibitors block the conversion of angiotensin I to angiotensin II. What does this result in?
    a. Instead of vasoconstriction, vasodilation occurs.
    b. Instead of vasodilation, vasoconstriction occurs.
    c. β-Adrenergic receptors are blocked, causing vasodilation.
    d. α-Adrenergic receptors are blocked, causing vasodilation.

18. Indicate whether each of the following statements regarding nursing care of the child with heart failure is true or false.
    a. **T F** The radial pulse is always taken before administering digoxin.
    b. **T F** Because infants with heart failure tire easily and may sleep through feedings, smaller feedings every 3 hours are often indicated.
    c. **T F** A fall in the serum potassium level enhances the effects of digitalis, decreasing the risk of digoxin toxicity.
    d. **T F** Infants and children should be positioned in at least a 45-degree angle to increase chest expansion.
    e. **T F** Infants should be fed on a 4-hour schedule to decrease fatigue.
    f. **T F** Sodium-restricted diets are used in children.
    g. **T F** Cyanosis is apparent when oxygen saturation is 80% to 85%.
    h. **T F** Patients with severe hypoxemia may exhibit fatigue with feeding, poor weight gain, tachypnea, and dyspnea.

Nursing Care of the Family and Child with Congenital Heart Disease

19. Mothers, fathers, and siblings are all affected when a child is diagnosed with a serious heart defect. Which of the following is correct?
    a. Mothers frequently feel adequate in their mothering ability because they often educate themselves by searching for the disorder online.
    b. Siblings typically feel included and closer to the family.
    c. Fathers often feel the need to be highly educated about the disorder.
    d. Mothers frequently feel inadequate in their mothering ability because of the more complex care infants with congenital heart defects require.

20. Identify four major nursing interventions that are included after cardiac surgery.
    a.

    b.

    c.

    d.

Acquired Cardiovascular Disorders

21. **T F** The most common causative agents are *Staphylococcus aureus* and *Streptococcus viridans*.

22. Prevention of bacterial endocarditis involves the administration of _____ therapy before procedures known to increase the risk of entry of organisms in very high–risk patients.
    a. vitamin C
    b. antibiotic
    c. antiviral
    d. antiseptic

23. _____ is a poorly understood inflammatory disease that occurs after infection with group A beta-hemolytic streptococcal pharyngitis.

182

Chapter **23** **The Child with Cardiovascular Dysfunction**

24. What can occur if strep throat is untreated?
    a. Bacterial meningitis
    b. Infectious mononucleosis
    c. Acute rheumatic fever
    d. Viral meningitis

25. Describe the following terms.
    a. Low-density lipoproteins (LDLs)

    b. High-density lipoproteins (HDLs)

26. The nurse is caring for an 8-year-old child just diagnosed with high cholesterol. What is the first step in the treatment plan for this child?
    a. Daily body weight measurement
    b. Medication administration and education
    c. Lifestyle modification interventions
    d. Weekly blood pressure checks

27. Which of the following patients with high cholesterol would be a good candidate for pharmacologic therapy?
    a. An 8-year-old child who has an LDL cholesterol greater than 190 mg/dl without other risk factors
    b. An 9-year-old child with an LDL cholesterol greater than 180 mg/dl without other risk factors
    c. An 11-year-old child with an LDL cholesterol greater than 180 mg/dl without other risk factors
    d. A 10-year-old child with an LDL cholesterol greater than 190 mg/dl without other risk factors

28. Which of the following is the treatment for atrioventricular blocks?
    a. Medications
    b. Pacemaker
    c. Vagal maneuvers
    d. Synchronized cardioversion

29. What disease is characterized by dyspnea with exercise, chest pain, and syncope?
    a. Pulmonary artery hypertension
    b. Dysrhythmia
    c. Atrioventricular blocks
    d. Sinus bradycardia

30. Which of the following diseases is characterized by abnormalities of the myocardium that impair the cardiac muscles' ability to contract?
    a. Atrioventricular blocks
    b. Pulmonary artery hypertension
    c. Cardiomyopathy
    d. Dysrhythmia

31. Anticoagulants may be given to reduce the risk of _____, a complication of the sluggish circulation through the heart.
    a. thromboemboli
    b. hypertension
    c. hypotension
    d. dysrhythmia

Heart Transplantation

32. Differentiate between an orthotopic and a heterotopic heart transplantation.

Vascular Dysfunction

33. What are the most common situations in which hypertension is observed in young children?

34. _____, or _____, is a complex clinical syndrome characterized by inadequate tissue perfusion to meet the body's metabolic demands, resulting in cellular dysfunction and eventual organ failure.

35. What three clinical manifestations result in circulatory failure in children?
    a.

    b.

    c.

36. Identify the three major goals of the therapeutic management of shock.
    a.

    b.

    c.

37. What does anaphylaxis result from?

A. Greg, 10 years old, is admitted to the pediatric unit for a cardiac catheterization the next morning. He and his parents appear anxious and uninformed.

   1. What should be included in the nursing assessment of Greg before the procedure?

   2. After the cardiac catheterization, Greg appears drowsy and has a pressure dressing on his right groin area. The most important nursing responsibility associated with the postprocedural care of Greg would be the detection of complications. Identify the rationale(s) for each of the following nursing interventions or observations.

      a. Taking frequent vital signs

      b. Monitoring blood pressure, especially for hypotension

      c. Assessing pulses distal to the catheterization site

      d. Assessing the temperature and color of the affected extremity

   3. What nursing intervention is appropriate to implement if bleeding occurs from the catheterization site?

B. Spend a day in an outpatient cardiac clinic to observe the nurse's role in the proper administration and evaluation of digoxin treatment.

   1. Describe the nurse's responsibility in administering digoxin.

   2. Why is the apical rate taken in a patient being treated with digoxin?

   3. Why must the nurse maintain a high index of suspicion for signs of toxicity when administering digoxin?

C. The nurse is caring for a hospitalized child with congestive heart failure.
  1. Why would a child with congestive heart failure be placed on a regimen of oral digitalis and diuretics?
     a. Digitalis

     b. Diuretics

  2. Why is it important for the nurse to monitor potassium levels in patients receiving potassium-losing diuretics and digoxin?

  3. What is a priority nursing diagnosis for the child with congestive heart failure?

  4. Identify two nursing interventions that can be used to help meet the goal of "Patient will exhibit improved cardiac output."
     a.

     b.

  5. Identify at least one expected outcome to the priority nursing diagnosis.

D. Demi, age 5, has just been diagnosed with coarctation of the aorta. Answer the following questions regarding nursing care of the family and child with congenital heart disease.
  1. When does nursing care of the child with a congenital heart defect begin?

  2. Explain the best approach the nurse would use to deal with the issue of the child's overdependence as a result of parental fear that their child may die.

  3. What should be included when educating the family about the child's cardiac disorder?

  4. What should the nurse tell the family regarding usage of the Internet as a source of information about heart disease in children?

E. Katie, age 14, comes into the emergency department. Immediately after eating strawberry jam, she started to feel uneasy, restless, dizzy, and disoriented. Her mother rushed her to the local hospital's emergency department. On assessment, the nurse notes hives on her face and neck, and urticaria. She is not having respiratory difficulty at this time.

  1. What is the possible cause of these clinical manifestations?

  2. What is the treatment of choice since she is not manifesting respiratory difficulty at this time?

  3. When anaphylaxis is suspected, what is the priority nursing intervention?

24 The Child with Hematologic or Immunologic Dysfunction

Chapter 24 introduces nursing considerations essential to the care of the child experiencing hematologic or immunologic dysfunction. The disorders discussed in this chapter are inherited, chronic, or terminal in nature and can result in extensive systemic and structural responses within the body. After completing this chapter, the student will be prepared to formulate a family-centered nursing care plan for the child with a hematologic or immunologic disorder.

REVIEW OF ESSENTIAL CONCEPTS

Hematologic and Immunologic Dysfunction

1. What four symptoms may be reported from a parent concerning the child's health history suggesting hematologic dysfunction?

    a.

    b.

    c.

    d.

2. A term used when describing an abnormal complete blood count (CBC) is _____, which refers to the presence of immature neutrophils in the peripheral blood from hyperfunction of the bone marrow.

3. _____ is the most common hematologic disorder of infancy and childhood. Although it is not a disease itself, it is an indication or manifestation of an underlying pathologic process.

4. Name and explain the two ways anemias are classified.

    a.

    b.

5. **T   F**   The basic physiologic defect caused by anemia is a decrease in the blood's oxygen-carrying capacity and consequently a reduction in the amount of oxygen available to the cells.

6. The following are suggested explanations for teaching children about blood components. Match each term with its defining characteristic.

    a. _____ Red blood cells

    b. _____ White blood cells

    c. _____ Platelets

    d. _____ Plasma

    1. Help keep germs from causing infection
    2. Small parts of cells that help make bleeding stop by forming a clot or scab over the hurt area
    3. The liquid part of blood that has clotting factors to help make bleeding stop
    4. Carry the oxygen you breathe from your lungs to all parts of your body

7. To assess and interpret laboratory studies for integration into a patient assessment, the nurse must understand the following laboratory measures. Identify the average value for each test, along with what each test measures.
   a. Red blood cell (RBC) count
   b. Hemoglobin (Hgb)
   c. Hematocrit (Hct)
   d. White blood cell (WBC) count
   e. Platelet count

Red Blood Cell Disorders

8. Why are children 12 to 36 months of age at risk for anemia?

9. An essential nursing responsibility is instructing parents in the administration of iron. How would the nurse instruct parents to administer oral iron to their child?

10. What is the objective of the medical management of anemia?

11. If the hemoglobin level fails to rise after 1 month of oral therapy, it is important to assess what five factors?
    a.

    b.

    c.

    d.

    e.

12. Iron stores in full-term infants are usually adequate for the first _____ to _____ months.

13. Packed red blood cells (RBCs), not whole blood, are given during transfusions for the most severe cases of anemia to minimize the chance of _____.

14. What are some side effects of oral iron therapy?

15. Describe the teaching interventions regarding iron supplementation that the nurse should provide in the following situations.
    a. Families of breastfed babies

    b. Families of formula-fed babies

16. Why should parents be instructed to keep no more than one month's supply of supplemental iron in the home?

17. The clinical features of sickle cell anemia (SCA) are primarily the result of what three factors?
    a.

    b.

    c.

18. Define *sickle cell trait*.

19. Identify the four types of sickle cell crisis.
    a.

    b.

    c.

    d.

20. Because early identification of SCA is essential, the _____ test is used for screening and case-finding; however, _____ is necessary to distinguish between children with the trait and those with the disease.

21. Identify the two major aims of the therapeutic management of SCA.
    a.

    b.

22. **T   F**   Oxygen administration reverses sickling of red blood cells.

23. What therapeutic treatment can result in depression of bone marrow, which further aggravates the anemia found in patients with SCA?

24. What complication would you consider in a patient with sickle cell disease (SCD) who presents with chest pain, fever, cough, and tachypnea?

25. Why is treatment important for SCD children who have experienced a stroke?

26. Match the following terms with the appropriate characteristic

    a. _____ Thalassemia minor   1. Produces a mild microcytic anemia
    b. _____ Thalassemia trait   2. Severe anemia requiring transfusion support
                                            3. Asymptomatic
    c. _____ Thalassemia intermedia   4. Moderate to severe anemia with splenomegaly
    d. _____ Thalassemia major

27. What are three other features of β-thalassemia outside of anemia?
    a.

    b.

    c.

28. What is the objective of supportive therapy in managing thalassemia?

29. What is one potential complication of frequent blood transfusions?

30. Oral or parenteral _____ are medications used to minimize the development of hemosiderosis.

31. Because of the risk of sepsis in a child with asplenia, what symptom should the family be told to notify the health professional if it arises?

32. List the onset of clinical manifestations in aplastic anemia.
   a.

   b.

   c.

33. A definitive diagnosis of aplastic anemia is determined from a _____ .

Defects in Hemostasis

34. _____ refers to a group of bleeding disorders in which there is a deficiency of one of the factors necessary for coagulation of the blood.

35. What are the two most common forms of hemophilia?
   a.

   b.

36. List the four objective signs of hemarthrosis.
   a.

   b.

c.

d.

37. What is the primary treatment for hemophilia?

38. What special precautions should health personnel use to prevent bleeding in patients with hemophilia?
    a.

    b.

    c.

39. What interventions should be implemented for a bleeding episode in a patient with hemophilia?
    a.

    b.

40. Identify the three factors that characterize idiopathic thrombocytopenic purpura (ITP).
    a.

    b.

    c.

41. A diagnosis of ITP is based on the platelet count being less than _____. Treatment is primarily

    _____.

42. Disseminated intravascular coagulation (DIC) is known as _____.

43. What are the three characteristics of DIC?
    a.

Chapter **24** **The Child with Hematologic or Immunologic Dysfunction**

b.

c.

44. Hallmarks of DIC are _____ and _____ that occur simultaneously.

45. Treatment of DIC is directed toward what?

Immunologic Deficiency Disorders

46. The human immunodeficiency virus (HIV) is a retrovirus transmitted by _____ and _____.

47. What are the two major pathways through which children acquire HIV?
    a.

    b.

48. Identify common clinical manifestations of HIV in children.
    a.

    b.

    c.

    d.

    e.

    f.

    g.

49. What is the cause, therapeutic management, and prognosis of acquired immune deficiency syndrome (AIDS)?
    a. Cause

    b. Therapeutic management

    c. Prognosis

50. What prevention factors should be included in educating all adolescents about HIV?

51. Severe combined immunodeficiency disease (SCID) is a defect characterized by an absence of both _____ and _____ immunity.

52. List common characteristics of SCID.
    a.

    b.

    c.

    d.

53. What is the only definitive treatment for SCID?

54. Wiskott-Aldrich syndrome (WAS) is a(n) _____ recessive disorder.

55. At birth, the presenting symptoms may be _____ or _____ as a result of thrombocytopenia.

Technologic Management of Hematologic and Immunologic Disorders
56. What types of immediate reactions can occur as the result of a blood transfusion?
    a.

    b.

c.

d.

e.

f.

g.

57. _____ is the removal of blood from an individual, separation of the blood into its components, retention of one or more of these components, and reinfusion of the remainder of the blood into the individual.

APPLYING CRITICAL THINKING TO THE NURSING PRACTICE

A. Regan, age 1 year, is admitted to the pediatric unit. In obtaining the neonatal and infant history, the nurse discovers that Regan was born 6 weeks prematurely. The nurse also discovers from the family history that Regan seemed to have excessive cow's milk ingestion over the past 2 months. On physical assessment, it is noted that Regan appears underweight and small for her age. Her family participates in the Women, Infants, and Children (WIC) program.

1. To determine the underlying condition, Regan will undergo a variety of blood tests. What nursing interventions can help prepare Regan and her family for these tests?

    a.

    b.

    c.

2. What factors put Regan at risk for iron-deficiency anemia?

3. A primary nursing objective is to use family education to prevent nutritional anemia. What information would be important for the nurse to explain to this family about preventing nutritional anemia?

B. Alicia, age 6, is hospitalized with sickle cell anemia. The nurse records her pain as 5 on the FACES pain scale (0–10). On physical assessment, it is noted that Alicia has a fever, cough, hematuria, tachypnea, and swollen extremities. Alicia is in a vaso-occlusive sickle cell crisis.

1. Describe two nursing diagnoses appropriate for Alicia.

   a.

   b.

2. Describe the most common pain control measure for managing severe pain during an SCA crisis. Include the medication regimen, along with specific pain medications used to treat SCA pain.

3. Alicia's parents are worried about addiction to pain medicine. What information could the nurse give this family about this concern?

C. Ryan, age 5, has hemophilia A and is being treated for bleeding.

1. What are the typical characteristics of this disorder?

   a.

   b.

2. What is the primary objective of treatment?

3. Ryan's nurse is going to perform a finger stick to obtain blood samples for the laboratory testing ordered by the physician. Should you allow the nurse to perform the finger stick? Why or why not?

4. Ryan's parents want to Ryan to remain active. What types of physical activities can the nurse encourage Ryan to do?

D. Dan, age 6 months, is being treated for AIDS.

1. What information concerning transmission should be discussed with Dan's parents?

   a.

   b.

   c.

Chapter **24** **The Child with Hematologic or Immunologic Dysfunction**

2. Should Dan receive his scheduled immunizations?

3. List at least three nursing diagnoses for Dan and his family.
   a.

   b.

   c.

The Child with Cancer

Chapter 25 introduces nursing considerations essential to the care of the child with a cancer diagnosis. The diseases discussed in this chapter include cancers of blood and lymph systems, nervous system tumors, bone tumors, and other solid tumors. After completing this chapter, the student will be prepared to formulate a family-centered nursing care plan for the child with cancer.

REVIEW OF ESSENTIAL CONCEPTS

Etiology

1. What factors predispose children to cancer?
   a.

   b.

   c.

2. **T F** Exposure to immunosuppressive therapy is a risk factor for cancer in children.

3. **T F** Lifestyle-related behaviors have little to no effect on childhood cancer.

4. What factors have significantly increased the survival rates for children with cancer?
   a.

   b.

   c.

Treatment Modalities

5. Chemotherapy agents can be classified according to their _____.

6. A potentially fatal complication of some chemotherapy agents is _____ and is characterized by _____.

7. How do biologic response modifiers alter the relationship between tumor and host?

8. Who are candidates for bone marrow transplantation?

a.

b.

Pediatric Oncologic Emergencies

9. **T F** The hallmark metabolic abnormalities of tumor lysis syndrome include hypouricemia, hypercalcemia, hypophosphatemia, and hypokalemia.

10. What are four risk factors for tumor lysis syndrome?

a.

b.

c.

d.

11. _____ is defined as a peripheral white blood cell count greater than $100,000/mm^3$.

12. Space-occupying lesions located in the chest may cause _____ and lead to _____ compromise and _____ failure.

13. What is the most common symptom in children with spinal cord compression?

Managing Side Effects of Treatment

14. A child with a fever who has an absolute neutrophil count lower than $500/mm^3$ is at risk for what three issues?

a.

b.

c.

15. What supportive measure is administered to prevent side effects caused by low blood counts?

16. How are most bleeding episodes prevented or controlled?

17. What activities should children at home who have low platelet counts avoid?

18. Blood transfusion with _____ may be necessary to raise the hemoglobin to appropriate levels.

19. What is the most beneficial regimen for the control of nausea and/or vomiting?

20. What supportive measures can the nurse promote in children with altered nutrition?

21. **T F** Lemon glycerin swabs are effective supportive measures for children with oral ulcers.

22. **T F** A satisfactory method of cleaning gums in infants and toddlers is to wrap a piece of gauze around a finger, soak it in saline, and swab the gums, palate, and inner check surfaces.

23. What is the most severe neurotoxic effect?

24. What neurologic syndrome may develop 5 to 8 weeks after central nervous system (CNS) radiation? How long does it typically last?

25. How can hemorrhagic cystitis be prevented?
    a.

    b.

    c.

    d.

26. What are two measures that can lessen the trauma of alopecia?

    a.

    b.

27. Why are children undergoing bone marrow transplant hospitalized for several weeks?

Health Promotion

28. **T F** Dental complications of children who received radiation to the head and neck include caries, periodontal disease, and facial asymmetry.

29. **T F** The child receiving chemotherapy for cancer should receive all immunizations as scheduled, including live, attenuated vaccines.

30. What two medications can be administered to a child receiving chemotherapy who has been exposed to the varicella virus in the past 2 days?

    a.

    b.

31. On what topics should the nurse educate the parent and child with cancer regarding home care?

Cancers of the Blood and Lymph System

32. What are the two major types of leukemia?

    a.

    b.

33. Leukemia is an unrestricted proliferation of _____ in the body's blood-forming tissues.

34. List the three main consequences of bone marrow dysfunction.

    a.

    b.

    c.

35. What are the most important prognostic factors in determining long-term survival for children with acute lympho-blastic leukemia?

36. A definitive diagnosis of leukemia is based on what diagnostic test(s)?

37. List the phases of chemotherapeutic therapy for leukemia.
    a.

    b.

    c.

38. Complete remission occurs with the presence of less than _____ blast cells in the bone marrow.

39. Why do children with leukemia receive CNS prophylactic therapy?

40. Differentiate between Hodgkin disease and non-Hodgkin lymphoma.
    a. Hodgkin disease

    b. Non-Hodgkin lymphoma

41. What is the most common presentation of Hodgkin disease?

Nervous System Tumors
42. Signs and symptoms of brain tumors are directly related to what two factors?
    a.

    b.

43. What is the treatment of choice for brain tumors?

44. What signs may indicate increased intracranial pressure and potential brainstem herniation?

45. Why is monitoring the temperature important in a postoperative child with a brain tumor?

46. _____ is the most common extracranial solid tumor of childhood and the most common cancer diagnosed in infancy.

47. Identify the stage of neuroblastoma with the characteristic.

a. _____ Stage 1

b. _____ Stage II (A or B)

c. _____ Stage III

d. _____ Stage IV

e. _____ Stage IV-S

1. Localized primary tumor with dissemination limited to the liver, skin, or bone marrow
2. Unilateral tumor with or without complete gross excision
3. Localized tumor confined to the area of origin and capable of complete gross excision
4. Tumor infiltrating across the midline with or without regional lymph node involvement
5. Dissemination of tumor to distant lymph nodes, bone, bone marrow, liver, skin, and other organs

Bone and Soft-Tissue Tumors

48. The peak age for pediatric bone tumors is _____ years and occurs more often in _____.

49. What bones are typically involved with the following bone cancers:
    a. Ewing sarcoma

    b. Osteosarcoma

50. If an amputation is performed for osteogenic sarcoma, the child may be fitted with a temporary _____ immediately after surgery.

51. Describe characteristics of phantom limb pain.

204

52. What is the treatment of choice for Ewing sarcoma?

53. What are the common presenting signs and symptoms for a child with a Wilms tumor?

54. Why is it important not to palpate the abdomen in a child with a Wilms tumor?

55. What are the three main nursing objectives in care of the child with a rhabdomyosarcoma?
    a.

    b.

    c.

56. Leukokoria or the cat's eye reflex is indicative of what diagnosis?

APPLYING CRITICAL THINKING TO THE NURSING PRACTICE

A. Dave, age 5, is hospitalized with a diagnosis of leukemia.
   1. What patient goal is appropriate for the nursing diagnosis "Risk for Infection"?

   2. List at least four nursing interventions appropriate for achieving this goal.
      a.

      b.

      c.

      d.

B. Janet is scheduled to receive L-asparaginase today for treatment of her acute lymphoblastic leukemia.
  1. What equipment should Janet's nurse have readily available?

  2. During Janet's infusion, she develops urticaria, flushing, nausea, and reports difficulty breathing.
     a. What is causing these symptoms?

     b. What should be done for Janet?

C. Ethan is 8 years old and recently was diagnosed with an infratentorial brain tumor. He had a partial resection of his tumor yesterday and is now postoperative day one.
  1. What areas of the neurologic assessment are important to monitor?

  2. What considerations should be taken when turning Ethan in bed?

  3. What interventions can the nurse perform to relieve Ethan's headache?

  4. Ethan is asking about the outcome of the surgery. What can the nurse say?

D. Katie is a 15-year-old adolescent diagnosed with osteosarcoma. She is scheduled for an amputation tomorrow.
  1. What should the nurse tell Katie to prepare her for the surgery?

  2. Katie is concerned about phantom limb pain. What interventions are available to help her with the pain after her surgery?

26 | The Child with Genitourinary Dysfunction

Chapter 26 introduces the nursing considerations essential to the care of the child who is experiencing genitourinary dysfunction. After completing this chapter, the student will be equipped with knowledge on nursing care of the child with common disorders of renal function, various types of diagnostic tests, renal dialysis, and transplantation. The student can use this knowledge to provide family-centered nursing care to the child with genitourinary dysfunction.

REVIEW OF ESSENTIAL CONCEPTS

Genitourinary Dysfunction

1. In the newborn, renal abnormalities may be associated with a number of other malformations. Which of the following malformations are most commonly associated with renal abnormalities in infants?
   a. Congenital heart conditions and abnormal shape or position of the outer ear
   b. Neural tube defects and abnormal shape or position of the inner ear
   c. Congenital heart conditions and abnormal shape or position of the inner ear
   d. Neural tube defects and abnormal shape or position of the outer ear

2. The single most important diagnostic laboratory test to detect renal problems is the _____.

3. Match each of the following urine tests of renal function with its purpose or significance of deviation.

   a. _____ Blood urea nitrogen
   b. _____ Specific gravity
   c. _____ Urine culture and sensitivity
   d. _____ Appearance
   e. _____ pH
   f. _____ Creatinine

   1. Determines the presence of pathogens and the drugs to which they are sensitive
   2. Normal result: 1.016 to 1.022; reflects the state of hydration
   3. Normal result of urine: newborn 5 to 7; thereafter, 4.8 to 7.8
   4. Newborn: 4 to 18; infant, child: 5 to 18
   5. Normal result: clear, pale yellow to deep gold
   6. Infant: 0.2 to 0.4; child: 0.3 to 0.7; adolescent: 0.5 to 1.0

Genitourinary Tract Disorders and Defects

4. What organism is the most common uropathogen for urinary tract infections (UTIs) in children?
   a. *Pseudomonas aeruginosa*
   b. *Escherichia coli*
   c. *Klebsiella*
   d. *Proteus mirabilis*

5. A 7-year-old girl presents with a UTI. What clinical manifestations of a UTI are common to this age group?
   a. Painful urination, swelling of face, pallor, blood in urine, and abdominal or back pain
   b. Excessive thirst, painful urination, pallor, blood in urine, and abdominal or back pain
   c. Failure to gain weight, swelling of face, pallor, blood in urine, abdominal or back pain
   d. Poor feeding, swelling of face, pallor, blood in urine, abdominal or back pain

6. List the four objectives of the therapeutic management of the child with a UTI.

   a.

   b.

   c.

   d.

7. **T F** Reflux causes febrile UTI.

8. Children with vesicoureteral reflux are very symptomatic. List some of the common symptoms they often display.

   a.

   b.

   c.

9. Indicate whether each of the following statements is true or false.
   a. **T F** Hypertension is a common result of glomerulonephritis.
   b. **T F** Urinary tract infections are commonly seen in patients with obstructive uropathy.

10. Indicate whether each of the following statements is true or false.
   a. **T F** The hazard of progressive renal injury is greatest when infection occurs in older children.
   b. **T F** Prevention is the most important goal in both primary and recurrent infection.
   c. **T F** Hydronephrosis occurs when interference with urine flow leads to a backup of urine.
   d. **T F** Hypospadias is where the urethral opening is located on the dorsal surface of the penis.

Glomerular Disease

11. A child presents with massive proteinuria, hypoalbuminemia, hyperlipidemia, and edema. Which of the following conditions are these symptoms associated with?
   a. UTI
   b. Ascites
   c. Nephrotic syndrome
   d. Acute glomerulonephritis

12. What is the hallmark of minimal-change nephrotic syndrome?
   a. Hyaline casts in the urine
   b. Massive proteinuria
   c. Oval fat bodies in the urine
   d. Large amounts of red blood cells in the urine

13. List the four objectives of the therapeutic management of nephrotic syndrome.

    a.

    b.

    c.

    d.

14. List four common side effects of steroid therapy in children.

    a.

    b.

    c.

    d.

15. Which of the following symptoms are commonly associated with acute poststreptococcal glomerulonephritis?
    a. Oliguria, edema, hypotension and circulatory congestion, hematuria, and proteinuria
    b. Oliguria, edema, hypertension and circulatory congestion, ascites, and proteinuria
    c. Oliguria, edema, hypotension and circulatory congestion, ascites, and proteinuria
    d. Oliguria, edema, hypertension and circulatory congestion, hematuria, and proteinuria

16. **T   F**   A child with acute poststreptococcal glomerulonephritis who presents with hypertension and edema does not need to be placed on a diet with moderate sodium restriction and even fluid restriction.

Miscellaneous Renal Disorders

17. Which of the following disorders has clinical manifestations of acquired hemolytic anemia, thrombocytopenia, renal injury, and central nervous system symptoms?
    a. Hydronephrosis
    b. Glomerular disease
    c. Hemolytic uremic syndrome
    d. Nephritic syndrome

18. What is the primary site of injury in hemolytic uremic syndrome?
    a. Red blood cells and fibrin clots
    b. Endothelial lining of the small glomerular arterioles
    c. Endothelial lining of the large glomerular arterioles
    d. Platelets and fibrin clots

19. What are the two goals of therapy for hemolytic uremic syndrome?

a.

b.

Renal Failure

20. Define the following terms.

a. Azotemia

b. Uremia

21. What is the principal feature of acute renal failure?
a. Polyuria
b. Dysuria
c. Oliguria
d. Hematuria

22. Which of the following is the baseline treatment of poor perfusion resulting from dehydration?
a. Blood transfusion
b. Sodium restricted diet
c. Fluid overload
d. Volume restoration

23. What is the most immediate threat to a child in acute renal failure?
a. Hyperkalemia
b. Hypercalcemia
c. Hypernatremia
d. Hypertension

24. A child presents to the hospital with symptoms of loss of normal energy, increased fatigue on exertion, and subtle pallor. The child states he has a headache, muscle cramps, and nausea. The child's mother states she has noticed slight bruising and swelling around his eyes and mouth. What do these symptoms suggest?
a. Late signs of chronic kidney disease
b. Early signs of chronic kidney disease
c. Early signs of acute renal failure
d. Late signs of acute renal failure

25. _____ is the most effective means, short of dialysis, for reducing the quantity of materials that require renal excretion.
a. Fluid restriction
b. Routine urinalysis
c. Daily labs
d. Diet regulation

Technologic Management of Renal Failure

26. List the three types of dialysis.
   a.

   b.

   c.

27. Which type of dialysis is preferred to preserve the child's independence?
   a. Hemodialysis
   b. Cycling dialysis
   c. Hemofiltration
   d. Peritoneal dialysis

28. A nurse is caring for an 8-year-old boy on dialysis and notes color of the dialysate is cloudy. What is the next step the nurse should take?
   a. Nothing. This is a normal and expected finding.
   b. Report this to the physician immediately.
   c. Remove the dialysate and start over.
   d. Check again in 4 hours and, if it's still cloudy, report the findings to the physician.

29. **T   F**   The preferred site for an arteriovenous fistula is the brachial artery and a hand vein.

30. Kidney _____ is now an acceptable and effective means of therapy in the pediatric age group.

APPLYING CRITICAL THINKING TO THE NURSING PRACTICE

A. Tami, age 4, is brought to the pediatrician by her mother, Nancy, who explains that, for the past few days, Tami has been wetting her bed at night and complaining of painful urination. In addition, just this morning, Tami ran a high temperature. Tami has also been complaining of not being hungry and frequently seems thirsty. A urine culture is obtained, and the pediatrician diagnoses Tami with a urinary tract infection (UTI).
   1. Which signs and symptoms of UTI should the nursing assessment yield?
      a.

      b.

      c.

      d.

      e.

2. What are the objectives of treatment for Tami?
   a.

   b.

   c.

   d.

3. What factors are considered when initiating antibiotic therapy for Tami?

4. What is the most important nursing goal when caring for children with UTIs?

B. Troy, age 5, is admitted to the acute pediatric floor. The nursing assessment reveals he has facial edema around his eyes, ascites, diarrhea, ankle and leg swelling, and lethargy. His parents report that he has been tired and irritable over the past week and that his clothes are fitting more tightly. They also report that he seems to be going to the bathroom less often than in the past.
1. What should Troy be evaluated for based on these clinical manifestations?

2. What would be an important nursing diagnosis related to the presence of edema in Troy?

3. What is the rationale for providing meticulous skin care?

4. The nurse must be cognizant that children on corticosteroid therapy are particularly vulnerable to what type of infection?

C. Tina, age 2, is admitted to the pediatric unit. Tina's history reveals that she has been vomiting, irritable, lethargic, and pale and has been bruising easily. Her mother reports she has also had bloody diarrhea.
   1. What do Tina's clinical manifestations suggest she might have?

   2. What is the most effective treatment for the identified condition?

   3. For the family to maintain home dialysis, the nurse must educate the family. What should be included in this teaching plan?
      a.

      b.

      c.

   4. Identify one nursing goal for Tina related to diet.

   5. What objective data could the nurse obtain to evaluate whether nursing interventions were successful in assisting Tina and her family with the stresses of chronic kidney disease?

D. The nurse is planning care for the child with chronic kidney disease.
   1. If the nursing diagnosis "Risk for Injury related to accumulated electrolytes and waste products" was chosen, what would be an appropriate patient goal?

   2. What are four appropriate nursing interventions for this nursing diagnosis?
      a.

      b.

      c.

      d.

27 The Child with Cerebral Dysfunction

Chapter 27 introduces the nursing considerations essential to the care of the child experiencing cerebral dysfunction. Dysfunction in the brain can produce alterations in the ways in which the child receives, integrates, and responds to stimuli. This chapter introduces the student to methods used to assess neurologic function in the unconscious child, along with methods to assess and intervene in the treatment of a child with cerebral trauma and seizure disorders. After completing this chapter, the student will be able to develop nursing goals and responsibilities that help the child and family effectively cope with the multiple stressors imposed by an alteration in cerebral function.

REVIEW OF ESSENTIAL CONCEPTS

Cerebral Dysfunction

1. Most information about infants and small children regarding their cerebral function is gained by observing their

   _____ and _____ responses. Persistence or reappearance of

   _____ that normally disappear indicates a pathologic condition.

2. What are the general aspects of assessment for cerebral dysfunction?
   a.

   b.

   c.

3. What are the signs and symptoms of increased intracranial pressure for infants and older children?
   a. Infants

   b. Children

4. What are some signs the nurse could expect to find in a child whose intracranial pressure becomes progressively worse?

5. Provide the name and explanation for the two components of consciousness.
   a.

   b.

6. _____ is defined as a state of unconsciousness from which the patient cannot be aroused, even with powerful stimuli.

7. Match the following terms that describe levels of consciousness with their defining characteristics.

a. _____ Disorientation

b. _____ Persistent vegetative state

c. _____ Full consciousness

d. _____ Obtundation

e. _____ Confusion

f. _____ Coma

g. _____ Stupor

h. _____ Lethargy

1. Awake and alert; orientated to time, place, and person; behavior appropriate for age
2. Decision making impaired
3. Inability to recognize the appropriate time and place; decreased level of consciousness
4. Limited spontaneous movement, sluggish speech, drowsiness
5. Arousable with stimulation
6. In a deep sleep and responsive only to vigorous and repeated stimulation
7. No motor or verbal response to noxious (painful) stimuli
8. Eyes following objects only by reflex; all four limbs spastic but can withdraw from painful stimuli

8. What three areas does the Glasgow Coma Scale assess?
   a.

   b.

   c.

9. Why is it essential that the neurologic examination be documented in a fashion that can be reproduced by others?

10. What pupil assessment would be considered a neurosurgical emergency?

11. How long does it take papilledema to develop in the early course of unconsciousness?

12. Define the types of posturing.
    a. Flexion posturing

    b. Extension posturing

Chapter **27** **The Child with Cerebral Dysfunction**

13. Three key reflexes that demonstrate neurologic health in young infants are the _____,

   _____, and _____ reflexes.

14. Because magnetic resonance imaging (MRI) can provoke anxiety in young children, sedation may be required.

   _____ or _____ has been used for years to sedate children for procedures such as MRI.

Nursing Care of the Unconscious Child

15. What four areas are the focus of emergency measures when caring for the unconscious child?
   a.

   b.

   c.

   d.

16. What signs could indicate pain in an unconscious child?

17. What are the four indications for inserting an intracranial pressure monitor?
   a.

   b.

   c.

   d.

Cerebral Trauma

18. Indicate whether each of the following statements is true or false.
   a. **T F** Falls are the major source of all head injuries in children between the ages of 0 to 14 years
   b. **T F** Because the head of an infant or toddler is proportionately larger and heavier in relation to other body parts, it is the least likely to be injured.
   c. **T F** Children with an acceleration/deceleration injury demonstrate diffuse generalized cerebral swelling produced by increased blood volume or a redistribution of cerebral blood volume (cerebral hyperemia) rather than by increased water content (edema), as seen in adults.

19. What are the hallmark symptoms of a concussion?

20. Define *contusions*.

21. Indicate whether each of the following statements is true or false.
    a. **T F** Clinically significant epidural hematomas are common in children younger than 2 years of age.
    b. **T F** Subdural hematomas are fairly common in infants, frequently as a result of birth trauma, falls, assaults, or violent shaking.
    c. **T F** Some degree of brain edema is expected after craniocerebral trauma, especially within 24 to 72 hours.
    d. **T F** Deep, rapid, periodic, or intermittent and gasping respirations; wide fluctuations or noticeable slowing of the pulse; and widening pulse pressure or extreme fluctuations in blood pressure are signs of temporal involvement.
    e. **T F** Computed tomography scan is the diagnostic test essential in diagnosing neurologic trauma.
    f. **T F** Bleeding from the nose or ears needs further evaluation, and a watery discharge from the nose (rhinorrhea) that is positive for glucose (as tested with Dextrostix) suggests leakage of cerebrospinal fluid (CSF) from a skull fracture.

22. What is the most important nursing observation in caring for a child with a head injury?

Submersion Injury

23. Match the age group with the common site for a submersion injury.

    a. _____ Infant younger than 1 year of age

    b. _____ Toddler

    c. _____ Preschooler

    d. _____ School-age child and adolescent

    1. Swimming pools
    2. Lakes, ponds, rivers
    3. Pail of liquid
    4. Bathtub

24. What are the major problems caused by submersion injuries?
    a.

    b.

    c.

25. What is the first priority in the therapeutic management of a submersion victim?

Chapter **27** **The Child with Cerebral Dysfunction**

Intracranial Infections

26. The nervous system is limited in the ways in which it responds to injury. If the inflammatory process affects the menin-

    ges, it is called _____; if it affects the brain, it is called _____.

27. The introduction of conjugate vaccines against _____ type b in 1990 and

    _____ in 2000 has led to the most dramatic change in the epidemiology of bacterial
    meningitis.

28. What organisms are responsible for the leading cases of bacterial meningitis in the following age groups?
    a. Neonates
    b. Children 3 months to 11 years
    c. Children 11 to 17 years

29. Indicate whether each of the following statements regarding bacterial meningitis is true or false.
    a. **T   F**   Pneumococcal and meningococcal infections can occur at any time but are more common in late winter
    or early spring.
    b. **T   F**   Invasion by direct extension from infections in the paranasal and mastoid sinuses is more common than
    invasion from an infection elsewhere in the body.
    c. **T   F**   There are no vaccines for bacterial meningitis.
    d. **T   F**   The onset of bacterial meningitis in children and adolescents is likely to be abrupt, with fever, chills,
    headache, and vomiting, and associated with or quickly followed by alterations in sensorium.

30. Why does a child who is ill and develops a purpuric or petechial rash need immediate medical attention?

31. List the interventions for the initial therapeutic management of acute bacterial meningitis.
    a.

    b.

    c.

    d.

    e.

    f.

    g.

h.

i.

32. Encephalitis can occur as a result of what two factors?
a.

b.

33. Treatment for encephalitis is primarily _____ and includes conscientious nursing care, control of cerebral manifestations, and adequate nutrition and hydration, with observation and management for other cerebral disorders.

34. Prognosis for the child with encephalitis depends on what three factors?
a.

b.

c.

35. _____ is transmitted to humans by the saliva of an infected mammal and is introduced through a bite or skin abrasion.

36. Current therapy for a rabid animal bite consists of what three interventions?
a.

b.

c.

37. Reye syndrome is a disorder defined as _____ associated with other characteristic organ involvement.

38. What are three clinical manifestations of Reye syndrome?
a.

b.

c.

39. There is a potential association between the use of _____ and the development of Reye syndrome.

40. Definitive diagnosis of Reye syndrome is established by _____.

Seizure Disorders

41. Seizures in children have many different causes. Seizures are classified according to _____

and _____.

42. Define *epilepsy*.

43. Identify and describe the two major categories of seizures.
    a.

    b.

44. A seizure occurs when there are what two conditions?
    a.

    b.

45. Identify 10 clinical entities that mimic seizures in children.
    a.

    b.

    c.

    d.

    e.

    f.

    g.

h.

i.

j.

46. _____ is obtained for all children with seizures and is the most useful tool for evaluating a seizure disorder. What does this test confirm?

47. What are the goals of the therapeutic management of seizures?
a.

b.

48. What is the primary therapy for seizure disorders?

49. How is the dosage of anticonvulsant drugs determined?

50. When anticonvulsant drugs are discontinued, what precautions should be taken?

51. The _____ diet has been shown to be an efficacious and tolerable treatment for medically refractory seizures.

52. When seizures are determined to be caused by a hematoma, tumor, or other cerebral lesion, _____ is the treatment.

53. _____ is a continuous seizure that lasts more than 30 minutes or a series of seizures from which the child does not regain a premorbid level of consciousness.

54. Why are children who have a single seizure not diagnosed with epilepsy and rarely started on antiepileptic drugs?

55. Children taking phenobarbital or phenytoin should receive adequate _____ and

_____ because deficiencies of both have been associated with these drugs.

56. List various seizure precautions.

57. _____ seizures are one of the most common seizure type, affecting approximately 2% to 5% of young children.

Cerebral Malformations

58. _____ is a condition caused by an imbalance in the production and absorption of CSF in the ventricular system, causing an increased accumulation of CSF in the ventricles.

59. What are the two results of hydrocephalus?
    a.

    b.

60. Hydrocephalus is so often associated with _____ that all infants with this condition should be observed for the development of hydrocephalus.

61. What are the most commonly observed clinical manifestations of hydrocephalus in the infant?
    a.

    b.

    c.

    d.

    e.

    f.

    g.

    h.

i.

j.

62. What is the typical treatment of hydrocephalus?

APPLYING CRITICAL THINKING TO THE NURSING PRACTICE

A. Tommy, age 6 months, was admitted to the pediatric unit after sustaining head trauma in an automobile accident. When admitted, he was conscious, but the nurse noted he had a bulging anterior fontanel, seemed irritable, had a high-pitched cry, and had distended scalp veins.
   1. What nursing diagnosis could be formulated from these assessment data?

   2. Tommy is becoming sleepy. When the nurse checked his pupils, they appeared fixed and dilated. What does this finding suggest?

B. Heather, age 10, has been unconscious for 2 days after surgery related to the trauma she endured from a motor vehicle accident.
   1. List signs of pain that Heather may demonstrate.
      a.

      b.

      c.

      d.

      e.

      f.

2. A patient goal is that Heather will exhibit no signs of pain. List three nursing interventions that could be used to achieve this goal.

a.

b.

c.

3. What parameters are assessed to monitor Heather's neurologic status?

a.

b.

c.

4. What nursing measure is taken to protect Heather's eyes from possible damage?

C. Spend a day in an emergency department for pediatric patients. Answer the following questions and include specifics (examples, responses) to illustrate these concepts.

1. Tara, age 2 years, sustained head trauma when she fell down some stairs. She was just admitted to the pediatric unit. The nurse notes a watery discharge from her nose. What is this nasal discharge called, and what does it suggest?

2. Sam, age 3 years, comes to the emergency department after being rescued from a swimming pool. What problems should the nurse recognize that could develop as a result of a submersion injury?

a.

b.

c.

D. Aden, age 8 months, is admitted to the pediatric unit with possible meningitis.

1. What clinical manifestations would you expect to assess in Aden?

2. What is a major priority of nursing care of a child with suspected meningitis?

E. Zach, age 6 years, was admitted to the pediatric unit for diagnosis and treatment of a possible seizure.
  1. What are the two major foci of the process of diagnosis in a child with a seizure disorder?
    a.

    b.

  2. While the nurse is assisting with breakfast, Zach has a brief loss of consciousness. The nurse noted that his eyelids twitched and his hands moved slightly. He then needed to reorient himself to previous activity. How would the nurse keep Zach safe?
    a.

    b.

    c.

    d.

    e.

    f.

F. Adam, a newborn, is transferred to the pediatric unit for treatment of hydrocephalus.
  1. What are some of the clinical manifestations of hydrocephalus?
    a.

    b.

    c.

    d.

    e.

    f.

2. List some of the postoperative nursing interventions for the newborn with hydrocephalus.

a.

b.

c.

d.

e.

f.

g.

h.

i.

j.

3. List the evaluative data that would indicate accomplishment of the following goal: The family will receive adequate education and emotional support.

28 The Child with Endocrine Dysfunction

Chapter 28 introduces the nursing considerations essential to the care of the child experiencing endocrine dysfunction. The conditions discussed in this chapter interfere with the body's ability to produce or respond to the major hormones. After completing this chapter, the student will be able to develop a nursing care plan to help provide family-centered care to the child with endocrine dysfunction.

REVIEW OF ESSENTIAL CONCEPTS

Disorders of Pituitary Function

1. _____ is a complex chemical substance produced and secreted into body fluids by a cell or group of cells that exerts a physiologic controlling effect on other cells.
   a. Glucose
   b. Blood pressure
   c. Hormone
   d. Adrenaline

2. The most common organic cause of pituitary undersecretion is
   a. autoimmune disease.
   b. excessive body weight.
   c. genetic disposition.
   d. tumor.

3. A nurse is caring for a child who presents with normal growth during the first year of life and then a slowed growth curve below the third percentile. What do these findings suggest?
   a. Normal for some children
   b. Growth hormone deficiency
   c. Hypothyroidism
   d. Hyperthyroidism

4. Why is it important to assess the parental history in children with constitutional growth delays?

5. What is the definitive treatment of growth hormone deficiency?

6. When is the best time to administer growth hormone?

7. A girl presents to the pediatric clinic with overgrowth of the head, lips, nose, tongue, jaw, and paranasal and mastoid sinuses; separation and malocclusion of the teeth in the enlarged jaw; disproportion of the face to the cerebral division of the skull; increased facial hair; and thickened, deeply creased skin. What do these clinical manifestations suggest?
   a. Acromegaly
   b. Diabetes insipidus
   c. Hyperthyrodism
   d. Hypermegaly

8. What is the primary nursing responsibility regarding hypopituitarism and hyperpituitarism?

9. Define *precocious puberty*.

10. The principal disorder of the posterior pituitary hypofunction is _____, which causes

    hyposecretion of antidiuretic hormone, producing a state of uncontrolled _____.

11. Identify the two cardinal signs of diabetes insipidus.
    a.

    b.

12. What is the usual treatment of diabetes insipidus?

13. What causes the syndrome of inappropriate antidiuretic hormone (SIADH)?

14. What is the immediate nursing management goal of SIADH?

Disorders of Thyroid Function

15. _____ is one of the most common endocrine problems of childhood.
    a. Type 1 diabetes
    b. Hypothyroidism
    c. Hyperthyroidism
    d. Metabolic compromise

16. What is the main physiologic action of the thyroid hormone?

17. Growth cessation or retardation in a child whose growth has previously been normal should alert the nurse to the

    possibility of _____.

18. A(n) _____ is an enlargement or "hypertrophy" of the thyroid gland.

19. _____ (also known as Hashimoto disease or _____) is the
    most common cause of thyroid disease in children and adolescents and accounts for the largest percentage of juve-
    nile hypothyroidism.

20. What is the most common cause of hyperthyroidism in children?
    a. Hypoparathyroidism
    b. Graves disease
    c. Addison disease
    d. Cushing syndrome

21. The clinical features of Graves disease in children consist of factors related to excessive motion. Identify at least
    three of the six factors.
    a.

    b.

    c.

22. Identify the three methods for treating Graves disease.
    a.

    b.

    c.

23. The most serious side effect of antithyroid drugs used to treat Graves disease is _____.

Disorders of Parathyroid Function

24. Identify the most common early symptom of hypoparathyroidism.
    a. Short stature
    b. Round face
    c. Seizures
    d. Muscle cramps

25. The diagnosis of hypoparathyroidism is made on the basis of clinical manifestations associated with decreased

    _____ and increased _____.

Disorders of Adrenal Function

26. Identify whether the following clinical manifestations are indicative of acute adrenocortical insufficiency or of hyperfunction of the adrenal gland (Cushing syndrome).
    a. Increased irritability, headache, diffuse abdominal pain, weakness, nausea and vomiting, diarrhea, fever, and central nervous system symptoms

    b. Centripetal fat distribution, "moon" face, muscular wasting, thin skin and subcutaneous tissue, poor wound healing, increased susceptibility to infection, decreased inflammatory response, excessive bruising, petechial hemorrhages, facial plethora, reddish purple abdominal striae, hypertension, hypokalemia, alkalosis, osteoporosis, hypercalciuria and renal calculi, psychoses, peptic ulcer, hyperglycemia, virilization, amenorrhea, and impotence

27. What should the nurse be alert to in the care and treatment of acute adrenocortical insufficiency in regard to the monitoring of electrolyte levels?

28. Cushing syndrome is a characteristic group of manifestations caused by excessive circulating free

    _____.

29. A characteristic sign of excess cortisol, whether from exogenous steroid therapy or a malfunction of the adrenal

    gland, is the _____ face.

30. A sex is assigned to the child with adrenogenital hyperplasia that is consistent with the _____,

    and _____ is administered to suppress the abnormally high secretions of adrenocorticotropic hormone.

31. What should parents have available when their infant is being treated with cortisol and aldosterone?

32. What causes the clinical manifestations of pheochromocytoma?

Disorders of Pancreatic Hormone Secretion: Diabetes Mellitus

33. What hormone is partially or completely deficient in diabetes mellitus?

34. When there is a deficiency in insulin, _____ cannot enter the cell.

35. Describe the two types of diabetes mellitus (DM), including the etiology of the disease processes.
    a. Type 1 diabetes mellitus

    b. Type 2 diabetes mellitus

36. Indicate whether each of the following statements is true or false.
    a. **T F** Acanthosis nigricans may be found in as many as 90% of children with type 2 diabetes and is characterized by velvety hyperpigmentation.
    b. **T F** Type 2 DM is the predominant form of diabetes in the pediatric age group, and type 1 diabetes is less common.
    c. **T F** Insulin is needed for the entry of glucose into the muscle and fat cells.
    d. **T F** When the glucose concentration in the glomerular filtrate exceeds the renal threshold (180 mg/dl), glucose spills into the urine (glycosuria), along with an osmotic diversion of water (polyuria), which is a cardinal sign of diabetes.
    e. **T F** Urinary fluid losses cause the excessive thirst (polydipsia) observed in diabetes.
    f. **T F** Without the use of carbohydrates for energy, fat and protein stores are replenished as the body attempts to meet its energy needs.
    g. **T F** Alteration in serum and tissue potassium can lead to cardiac arrest.
    h. **T F** Kussmaul respirations are characteristic of respiratory acidosis.

37. Identify the three principal microvascular complications of diabetes.
    a. Nephropathy, retinopathy, neuropathy
    b. Hypertension, nephropathy, retinopathy
    c. Hyperglycemia, retinopathy, neuropathy
    d. Nephropathy, retinopathy, excessive weight gain

38. Diabetes is a great imitator of what conditions?
    a. Influenza, hypothyroidism, appendicitis
    b. Influenza, gastroenteritis, appendicitis
    c. Influenza, hyperthyroidism, appendicitis
    d. Influenza, viral meningitis, appendicitis

39. What are the three "polys" of diabetes mellitus?
    a.

    b.

    c.

40. Diagnosis of diabetes can be obtained through an 8-hour fasting blood glucose level of _____ mg/dl or more, or a random blood glucose value of _____ mg/dl or more accompanied by classic signs of diabetes. An oral glucose tolerance test finding of _____ mg/dl or more in the 2-hour sample is almost certain to indicate diabetes.

41. Human insulin is packaged in the strength of 100 units/ml. Match each of the following types of insulin with the appropriate rate of action (peak effect).

a. _____ Neutral protamine Hagedorn

b. _____ Regular insulin

c. _____ NovoLog insulin

d. _____ Lantus insulin

1. Rapid-acting
2. Short-acting
3. Intermediate-acting
4. Long-acting

42. Match each of the following age groups with the appropriate target A_{1c} (%).

a. _____ Toddlers and preschoolers (>6 years)

b. _____ School age (6 to 12 years)

c. _____ Adolescents (>12 years) and young adults

1. <8%
2. ≤8.5% (but ≥7.5%)
3. <7.5%

43. _____ are designed to deliver fixed amounts of regular insulin continuously, thereby imitating the release of the hormone by the islet cells.

44. What has improved diabetes management and can be used successfully by children?

45. What does exercise do for the child with diabetes?

46. Describe the Somogyi effect and its treatment.

47. What are the most common causes of hypoglycemia?

48. A child with type 1 diabetes presents to the emergency room with sweating, hunger, weakness, dizziness, headache, drowsiness, irritability, and loss of coordination. What do these clinical manifestations suggest?
    a. Somogyi effect
    b. Hyperglycemia
    c. Hypoglycemia
    d. The immediate need for insulin

49. The appropriate emergency measure when a child with diabetes is having a hypoglycemic reaction is to administer

    _____ in some form.

50. Diabetic ketoacidosis is a state of medical emergency. The nurse must recognize that the priority is to obtain a

    _____ for administration of fluids, electrolytes, and insulin.

APPLYING CRITICAL THINKING TO THE NURSING PRACTICE

A. Spend a day in a pediatric endocrine clinic. Answer the following questions and include specific examples or responses to illustrate these concepts.
    1. What cardinal signs would the nurse expect to assess in a child with diabetes insipidus?
        a.

        b.

    2. What clinical manifestations would the nurse expect to assess in a child with hyperpituitarism before epiphyseal closure?
        a.

        b.

        c.

        d.

    3. What clinical manifestations of lymphocytic thyroiditis would the nurse expect to find?
        a.

        b.

        c.

    4. What physical signs would the nurse expect to see in the acute onset of a thyroid storm?
        a.

        b.

c.

d.

e.

f.

g.

h.

5. A nurse is caring for a child. Upon assessment, the nurse notes short stature; round face; short, thick neck; short, stubby fingers and toes; and dimpling of the skin over the knuckles. What do these clinical manifestations suggest?
   a. Pseudohypoparathyroidism
   b. Hypoparathyroidism
   c. Hypothyroidism
   d. Type 2 diabetes

B. The nurse is caring for a child with adrenocortical insufficiency. Answer the following questions and include specifics (examples, responses) to illustrate these concepts.
   1. During the neurologic assessment on admission, the nurse notes muscular weakness, mental fatigue, irritability, apathy, negativism, increased sleeping, and listlessness. Which type of adrenocortical insufficiency do these signs describe?

   2. After the nurse instructs the child's parents about the administration of cortisol to the child, what should the parents demonstrate regarding their understanding of cortisol and the dangers in stopping the medication?

   3. As treatment progresses, the nurse continually assesses the child for signs of hypokalemia. What are these signs?

C. The nurse is caring for a child with pheochromocytoma.
   1. What are at least five clinical manifestations that the nurse recognizes as being characteristic of pheochromocytoma?
      a.

      b.

c.

d.

e.

2. The nurse understands the palpation of the mass in the child with pheochromocytoma may lead to the release of

_____. What can these do?

D. Joe, a 10-year-old boy, is on the pediatric unit for diagnosis and treatment of diabetes mellitus.
   1. When Joe arrived on the unit, he had ketonuria and acetone breath. What emergency condition is he displaying?

   2. What is the definitive treatment for Joe's condition?

   3. Joe says he is "scared to death" of needles. Based on his stated fear, explain what would be the best approach to administering insulin to treat his newly diagnosed diabetes mellitus?

   4. What is the best method to determine the amount of insulin Joe will need to regulate his blood glucose?

   5. What should the nurse recognize as the cornerstone of diabetes management and the major responsibility in diabetes nursing care?

   6. After Joe's first week of insulin therapy, he plays a game of basketball. He starts to feel nervous and irritable. He notices he has difficulty concentrating on the game and is unable to focus on what he is doing. He begins to shake and sweat.
      a. What is Joe experiencing?

      b. Intervene to treat this experience. What measures could the nurse suggest to Joe to help prevent this occurrence from happening in future basketball games?

7. The nurse identifies the nursing diagnosis of "Risk for Injury related to hypoglycemia" for Joe. What are three interventions that will help Joe meet the patient goal of "Patient will exhibit no evidence of hypoglycemia"?

   a.

   b.

   c.

8. What is the expected outcome for this goal?

9. It is important for Joe and his parents to know that his blood sugar levels will be affected by illness. What should the nurse stress about the importance of taking insulin when Joe is ill?

29 The Child with Musculoskeletal or Articular Dysfunction

Chapter 29 introduces nursing considerations in the care of the child immobilized with an injury or a degenerative disease. The disorders considered are of congenital, acquired, traumatic, infectious, neoplastic, or idiopathic origin. On completion of this chapter, the student will be prepared to formulate nursing goals and interventions to provide family-centered care to the child with musculoskeletal or articular dysfunction.

REVIEW OF ESSENTIAL CONCEPTS

The Immobilized Child

1. What three factors cause most of the pathologic changes that occur during immobilization?
   a.

   b.

   c.

2. When does joint contracture begin during immobilization?

3. All children who are immobilized are at risk for skin breakdown. What three factors put some children at an even greater risk for skin breakdown?
   a.

   b.

   c.

Traumatic Injury

4. Define the following traumatic injuries.
   a. Contusion

   b. Dislocation

c. Sprain

d. Strain

5. The first minutes to 12 hours are the most critical period for virtually all soft-tissue injuries. Basic principles of managing sprains and other soft-tissue injuries are summarized in the acronyms RICE and ICES. What do these acronyms stand for?
a. RICE

b. ICES

6. Any investigation of fractures in infants, particularly multiple fractures, should include consideration of

_____.

7. If the fracture does not produce a break in the skin, it is a _____ or

_____ fracture. Fractures with an open wound through which the bone protrudes are

called _____ or _____ fractures.

8. What is the most effective diagnostic tool in assessing skeletal trauma?

9. **T   F**   Fractures heal in less time in children than in adults.

10. **T   F**   Spica casts are used to immobilize the spine.

11. What are the four goals of the therapeutic management of fractures?
a.

b.

c.

d.

12. Identify the six *P*s of ischemia from a vascular injury.

   a.

   b.

   c.

   d.

   e.

   f.

13. During the first few hours after a cast is applied, what is the chief concern about the extremity? How is this likelihood reduced?

14. Identify and describe the three essential components of traction management.

   a.

   b.

   c.

15. What factors determine the type of traction?

   a.

   b.

   c.

16. _____ is the process of separating opposing bone to encourage regeneration of new bone in the created space.

17. When amputated, a severed part should be preserved in what manner to facilitate reattachment?

Birth and Developmental Defects

18. Identify and describe the three broad categories of predisposing factors associated with developmental dysplasia of the hip (DDH)?
    a.

    b.

    c.

19. Why is radiographic examination in early infancy for DDH not reliable?

20. Match each type of clubfoot position with its defining characteristic.

    a. _____ Talipes varus   1. Toes lower than the heel and facing inward
                                         2. Plantar flexion, in which the toes are lower than the heel
    b. _____ Talipes equinus   3. An eversion, or bending outward
                                         4. Dorsiflexion, in which the toes are higher than the heel
    c. _____ Talipes valgus   5. An inversion, or bending inward

    d. _____ Talipes calcaneus

    e. _____ Talipes equinovarus

21. Therapeutic management of congenital clubfoot involves:
    a.

    b.

    c.

22. Deletion or shortening of digits or limbs may also be associated with _____, especially before 10 to 12 weeks of gestation; however, the incidence and relationship remain uncertain.

23. Osteogenesis imperfecta is a heterogeneous, autosomal dominant disorder characterized by

_____ and _____.

24. The goals of rehabilitative approach to management in children with osteogenesis imperfecta are directed toward preventing:
   a.

   b.

   c.

Acquired Defects
25. Describe the pathophysiology of Legg-Calvé-Perthes disease.

26. The aims of treatment of Legg-Calvé-Perthes disease include what four factors?
   a.

   b.

   c.

   d.

27. _____ refers to the spontaneous displacement of the proximal femoral epiphysis in a posterior and inferior direction.

28. Match the following deformities of the spine with the proper defining characteristics of that deformity.

   a. _____ Kyphosis   1. An accentuation of the cervical or lumbar curvature beyond physiologic limits
   b. _____ Lordosis   2. An abnormally increased convex angulation in the curvature of the spine
                              3. A lateral curvature and spinal rotation causing rib asymmetry
   c. _____ Scoliosis

29. How is scoliosis definitively diagnosed?

30. What are the main methods of management of scoliosis?

   a.

   b.

   c.

31. What conditions require surgical treatment?

Infections of Bones and Joints

32. _____ is an infectious process in the bone. It can occur at any age but is most frequently

   seen in children 10 years of age or younger. _____ is the most common causative
   organism.

33. Supporting evidence for the diagnosis of osteomyelitis includes what laboratory results?

34. When the infective agent of osteomyelitis is identified, vigorous _____ therapy is initi-

   ated with an appropriate _____.

35. What therapy is instituted to ensure restoration of optimum function after the infection resolves in a child with
   osteomyelitis?

Disorders of Joints

36. What is the new name replacing juvenile rheumatoid arthritis? Why was a new name given?

37. What are the major goals of therapy for the child with JIA?
   a.

   b.

   c.

   d.

38. What are the primary groups of drugs prescribed for JIA?
   a.

   b.

   c.

   d.

39. **T   F**   Practitioners may recommend nighttime splinting to help minimize pain and reduce flexion deformity.

40. **T   F**   Corticosteroids are the first drugs of choice for JIA.

41. **T   F**   Moist heat, such as a whirlpool bath, is beneficial to children with arthritis.

42. _____ is a chronic, multisystem, autoimmune disease of the connective tissues and blood vessels characterized by inflammation in potentially any body tissue.

43. Describe a characteristic cutaneous response of systemic lupus erythematosus (SLE).

44. Identify the principal drugs employed to control the inflammation of SLE.

45. The child with SLE and his or her family must learn to recognize subtle signs of _____

   and potential complications of _____, and to communicate these concerns to their health care provider.

A. Spend a day on the neurologic unit observing the care of immobilized children. On the unit, the nurse should plan the care of the immobilized child with the knowledge that immobilization causes functional and metabolic responses in most of the body's systems.
   1. What are the major musculoskeletal consequences of immobilization?

   2. What is the rationale for frequent position changes?

   3. What are some of the primary effects of immobilization on the cardiovascular system?

B. Billy, a 2-year-old child, comes into the after-hours care center with his father and mother. Billy's father said he was holding Billy's hand when they were walking down the stairs to leave the crowded football game. Billy began to try to pull and run away, so the father jerked tightly onto Billy's arm to keep him close. Billy cried, was anxious, and began holding his right arm. In the after-hours clinic, Billy is sitting and still bracing his arm.
   1. What type of injury did Billy probably sustain?

   2. How is this type of injury treated?

C. Kendra, a 10-year-old girl, is in 90-degree traction after a fall from a two-story building.
   1. List at least four ways skin breakdown is prevented in the child who is in traction.
      a.

      b.

      c.

      d.

   2. How is alignment maintained for the child who is in traction?
      a.

      b.

c.

D. The nurse is caring for a child with developmental dysplasia of the hip (DDH).
   1. During the infant assessment process, what clinical signs could indicate DDH in the newborn?
      a.

      b.

      c.

      d.

      e.

   2. How does the method of handling infants in various cultures relate to the development of dysplasia of the hip in the newborn?

   3. How is the hip joint maintained to promote normal hip development?

E. Jose, age 8 years, is admitted for treatment of osteogenesis imperfecta.
   1. What clinical manifestations would the nurse expect to find in Jose if the diagnosis is correct?

   2. What two things does the rehabilitative approach to management of osteogenesis imperfecta aim to prevent?
      a.

      b.

F. Tina, age 13 years, is admitted to the pediatric unit for treatment of JIA.
   1. The former drug of choice for treating JIA was aspirin. What class of drug has replaced aspirin as the drug of choice? Why was aspirin replaced?

Chapter **29** **The Child with Musculoskeletal or Articular Dysfunction**

2. How is JIA diagnosed?

3. Identify five nursing goals for treating Tina.
   a.

   b.

   c.

   d.

   e.

30 The Child with Neuromuscular or Muscular Dysfunction

Chapter 30 introduces nursing considerations essential to the care of the child with a disorder of neuromuscular function. The conditions discussed in this chapter may result from defective transmission of nerve impulses to muscles, dysfunction of peripheral motor or sensory nerves, or damage to the central nervous system. After completing this chapter, the student will be prepared to formulate nursing goals and interventions that provide family-centered care to the child with neuromuscular or muscular dysfunction.

REVIEW OF ESSENTIAL CONCEPTS

Congenital Neuromuscular or Muscular Disorders

1. Which of the following is most likely to develop cerebral palsy?
   a. A Caucasian female infant with a birth weight of 1330 grams at birth born at 27 weeks' gestation
   b. A Caucasian male infant with a birth weight of 1330 grams at birth born at 27 weeks' gestation
   c. An African American female infant with a birth weight of 1330 grams at birth born at 27 weeks' gestation
   d. An African American male infant with a birth weight of 1330 grams at birth born at 27 weeks' gestation.

2. Intrauterine exposure to maternal _____ is associated with an increased risk of cerebral palsy (CP) in infants of normal birth weight and preterm infants.

3. List the four classifications of CP, which are based on the nature and distribution of neuromuscular dysfunction.
   a.

   b.

   c.

   d.

4. What are the primary modalities for diagnosing CP?
   a. History and vital signs
   b. History and musculoskeletal examination
   c. History and magnetic resonance imaging
   d. History and neurologic examination

5. What are some physical warning signs that point toward possible CP early in life?
   a. Poor head control after 2 months of age
   b. Stiff or rigid neck
   c. Floppy or limp body posture
   d. Inability to sit up without support by 6 months of age

6. Identify the goals of therapeutic management for children with CP
   a. Early recognition and full range of motion
   b. Early recognition and promotion of optimal development
   c. Early recognition and medication administration
   d. Early recognition and physical therapy

7. What drug is used to decrease spasticity in children with CP?

8. What are five problems common among children with CP?
   a.

   b.

   c.

   d.

   e.

9. According to available data, approximately _____ of individuals with CP have cognitive impairments.
   a. 20% to 50%
   b. 10% to 60%
   c. 50% to 75%
   d. 30% to 50%

10. What form of spina bifida cystica encases meninges and spinal fluid but no neural elements?
    a. Meningocele
    b. Myelomeningocele
    c. Meningomyelocele
    d. Anencephaly

11. Which of the following is an important nursing intervention when caring for a child with a myelomeningocele in the preoperative stage?
    a. Applying a heat lamp to facilitate drying and toughening of the sac
    b. Assessing sensory and motor function frequently to monitor for signs of impairment
    c. Applying a diaper to prevent contamination of the sac
    d. Placing the child on his or her side to decrease pressure on the spinal cord

12. It has been estimated that a daily intake of _____ in women of childbearing age will prevent 50% to 70% of all cases of neural tube defects.
    a. 0.8 mg of folic acid
    b. 1 mg of folic acid
    c. 0.4 mg of folic acid
    d. 0.6 mg of folic acid

13. What are some symptoms of latex allergy in infants?
    a.

b.

c.

d.

e.

14. What are the important goals of therapy regarding latex allergy?
    a.

    b.

15. _____ disease is a disorder characterized by progressive weakness and wasting of skeletal muscles caused by degeneration of anterior horn cells. It is inherited as an autosomal recessive trait and is the most common paralytic form of the floppy infant syndrome (congenital hypotonia).

16. How is Werdnig-Hoffmann disease treated?

17. What is the most common form of muscular dystrophy?

18. What is the most common cause of death in Duchenne muscular dystrophy?

19. What is the primary goal of therapeutic management of muscular dystrophy?
    a. Prevention of contractures
    b. Prevention of infections
    c. Prevention of cognitive deficits
    d. Maintaining optimal function in all muscles for as long as possible

Acquired Neuromuscular Disorders
20. Define Guillain-Barré syndrome (GBS).

21. What are three of the eight initial symptoms of GBS?

a.

b.

c.

22. How is GBS treated?

23. Tetanus, or lockjaw, is an acute, preventable, but often fatal disease caused by an exotoxin produced by the anaerobic spore-forming, gram-positive bacillus _____.

24. Preventive measures for tetanus are based on the _____ of the affected child and the nature of the injury.

25. What is the treatment for the unimmunized child who sustains a tetanus-prone wound?

26. What causes infant botulism? Where are prime sources of botulism found?

27. What are some common symptoms of infant botulism?

a.

b.

c.

d.

28. What is the diagnosis of botulism based on?

29. How is infant botulism treated?

30. The most common cause of serious spinal cord damage in children is trauma involving _____.

31. Define the following terms.
   a. Paraplegia

   b. Quadriplegia

32. What three factors are the focus in the nursing management of spinal cord injury (SCI)?
   a.

   b.

   c.

33. During the recovery and rehabilitation phase, patients with SCI must be carefully monitored for complications of

   immobility, such as _____ and _____.

APPLYING CRITICAL THINKING TO THE NURSING PRACTICE

A. Angela, age 10 years, is being treated for problems related to cerebral palsy. Her biggest concern right now is her repeated injuries and accidents due to her physical disabilities.
   1. Identify the priority nursing diagnosis for Angela.

   2. What would a patient goal be for Angela related to this diagnosis?

   3. What are some nursing interventions the nurse could implement to meet this goal?
      a.

      b.

      c.

Chapter **30** **The Child with Neuromuscular or Muscular Dysfunction**

d.

e.

f.

4. Identify nursing interventions for Angela and her family.

B. Ada, a newborn, is transferred to the pediatric unit for surgical evaluation of a myelomeningocele.
  1. What are three nursing goals for Ada's initial care?
     a.

     b.

     c.

  2. What assessment data would indicate the accomplishment of each of the nursing goals identified in question 1?
     a.

     b.

     c.

C. Spend a day in a clinic that treats children with muscular dystrophy.
  1. What is the major emphasis of nursing care for a child with muscular dystrophy?

  2. What type of counseling is recommended for parents, sisters, and maternal aunts and their female offspring?

D. Tina, age 16 years, has been admitted to the pediatric unit with a diagnosis of Guillain-Barré syndrome (GBS).
  1. On what three factors is the diagnosis of GBS based?
     a.

b.

c.

2. What medication has been reported to be most effective in treating chronic neuropathic pain in GBS?

E. Jim, age 16 years, is hospitalized in a rehabilitation center for treatment of paraplegia caused by a spinal cord injury he sustained in a motor vehicle crash.
   1. Explain the physiologic trauma responsible for most spinal cord injuries in children.

   2. What is the major aim of Jim's physical rehabilitation?

Answer Key

CHAPTER 1

Review of Essential Concepts

1. c
2. b
3. d
4. a
5. c
6. d
7. a
8. b
9. d
10. The number of deaths per 1000 live births during the first year of life
11. b
12. b
13. c
14. a. Congenital anomalies
    b. Disorders relating to short gestation and unspecified low birth weight
    c. Sudden infant death syndrome
    d. Newborn affected by maternal complications of pregnancy
15. c
16. d
17. d
18. psychologic, physical
19. a. Prevent or minimize the child's separation from the family
    b. Promote a sense of control
    c. Prevent or minimize bodily injury and pain
20. therapeutic relationship
21. a
22. boundaries
23. d
24. b
25. b
26. c
27. d
28. a
29. b
30. c
31. a
32. It is a cognitive process that uses formal and informal thinking to gather and analyze patient data, evaluate the significance of the information, and consider alternative actions.
33. The nursing process is a method of problem identification and problem solving that describes what the nurse actually does.
    a. Assessment
    b. Diagnosis
    c. Planning
    d. Implementation
    e. Evaluation
34. a. 2
    b. 4
    c. 1
    d. 3
    e. 5
35. problem statement, etiology, signs and symptoms
36. a. 1
    b. 3
    c. 2
37. The degree to which health services for individuals and populations increase the likelihood of desired health outcomes and are consistent with current professional knowledge

Applying Critical Thinking to the Nursing Practice

A.

1. Ensure families' awareness of various health services; inform families of treatments and procedures; involve families in child's care; change or support existing health care practices.
2. Practice within the overall framework for preventive health; employ an approach of education and anticipatory guidance.
3. Provide continual assessment and evaluation of the child's physical, emotional, and developmental status.
4. Work with professionals in other disciplines to formulate and implement a care plan that meets the child's needs.
5. Determine the least harmful action within the framework of societal mores, professional practice standards, the law, institutional rules, religious traditions, the family's value system, and the nurse's personal values.
6. Conduct research to provide theoretical foundations for the nursing practice and to evaluate the nursing process.
7. Involve the family in all steps of the nursing process.

B.

1. Violated: Recognize that the family is the constant in a child's life. Consider the needs of the family members—not just the child. Work to extend family visitation hours. Cluster care in units that still have times when the unit is closed to visitors to provide the family with more meaningful interaction times with their child.
2. Violated: Family members, especially siblings, should have free access to their family member. Work to extend visitation hours and to allow siblings of any age to visit. If this is not possible, strive to have a viewing room so siblings can see their brother or sister.
3. Applied: Enabling family members to display their ability and competence fosters a parent-professional partnership. This could be enhanced by including the family members in scheduling activities of daily living throughout the day.
4. Applied: This empowers the family member to maintain a sense of control over daily activities. This intervention could be further enhanced by asking the mother what activities of daily living she would like to assist with or perform throughout the day during the initial morning assessment.

CHAPTER 2

Review of Essential Concepts

1. b
2. c

3. d
4. d
5. a
6. c
7. a. 7
   b. 6
   c. 5
   d. 4
   e. 3
   f. 2
   g. 1
8. b
9. c
10. authoritarian
11. a
12. b
13. c
14. a
15. c
16. a
17. d
18. d
19. b
20. Joint legal custody occurs when children reside with one parent but both parents are legal guardians and both participate in childrearing.
21. a. T
    b. T
    c. T
22. a. T
    b. F
    c. T
23. Bronfenbrenner
24. c
25. a. Young people need to feel support, care, and love from their families, neighbors, and others. They also need organizations and institutions that offer positive, supportive environments.
    b. Young people need to feel valued by their community and be able to contribute to others. They need to feel safe and secure.
    c. Young people need to know what is expected of them, what activities and behaviors are within the community boundaries, and what are outside of them.
    d. Young people need opportunities for growth through constructive, enriching opportunities and through quality time at home.

Applying Critical Thinking to the Nursing Practice

A.
1. a. Tasks include integrating infants into the family unit, accommodating to new parenting roles, and maintaining the marital bond.
   b. Children develop new peer relations and new roles. They also spend more time away from parents. Parental role changes include adjusting to children's peer and school relationships while maintaining the marital bond.
2. Parental age, father's involvement, parenting education, stressors in the family, having a child with a difficult temperament, stressed marital relationships, support systems

B.
1. Events such as marriage, divorce, birth, sickness, stressors (new sibling, career change, moving residences), financial stress, marital stress, lack of social support, death, abandonment, and incarceration
2. Roles must be redefined or redistributed.
3. a. Commitment
   b. Appreciation
   c. Time
   d. Purpose
   e. Congruence
   f. Communication
   g. Family rules, values, beliefs
   h. Coping strategies
   i. Problem solving
   j. Positive attitude
   k. Flexibility and adaptability
   l. Balance

C.
1. The parent may feel guilty about time spent away from children; overburdened by responsibility and demands on time; depressed and doubtful of ability to cope with the child's emotional needs; isolated and lonely; and overworked and anxious about the financial difficulties often associated with being a single-parent family.
2. a. Health care services that are open nights and weekends
   b. High-quality child care
   c. Respite child care
   d. Parent enhancement centers

D.
Examples of weaknesses of dual-career parents include less quality time spent with the children, more reported guilt, overload, stress, and undefined roles. Strengths of dual-career parents may include higher education levels of parents, better child care options, less isolation and loneliness, and fewer financial stressors. Examples of weaknesses of a family with a career parent and a stay-at-home parent include specific and somewhat fixed gender roles, less quality time to care for self, risk of isolation and loneliness, and more pressure and stress on the career parent. Strengths of families with a career parent and a stay-at-home parent include more defined roles, more social support from one another and often more support for the children, less hectic schedules throughout the work week, and more quality time for the children at home with a parent.

CHAPTER 3

Review of Essential Concepts

1. a. 3
   b. 1
   c. 2
   d. 4
2. quantitative, qualitative
3. d
4. b
5. The head end of the organism develops first and is very large and complex, whereas the lower end is small and simple and takes shape at a later period. The physical evidence of this trend is most apparent during the period before birth, but it also applies to postnatal behavior development. Infants achieve structural control of the head before they have control of the trunk and extremities, hold their back erect before they stand, use their eyes before their hands, and gain control of their hands before they have control of their feet.
6. Development is near-to-far or midline-to-peripheral. A conspicuous illustration is the early embryonic development of limb

buds, followed by rudimentary fingers and toes. In the infant, shoulder control precedes mastery of the hands, the whole hand is used as a unit before the fingers can be manipulated, and the central nervous system develops more rapidly than the peripheral nervous system.

7. Gross, fine
8. a. T
   b. F: Growth and development progress at different rates.
   c. F: It is the first three months.
9. a. 2
   b. 1
   c. 4
   d. 3
10. b
11. 4, 7, triples, quadruples
12. c
13. d
14. The tissues are small in relation to body size but are well developed at birth. They increase rapidly to reach adult dimensions by 6 years of age and continue to grow. At about age 10 to 12 years, they reach a maximum development approximately twice their adult size. This is followed by a rapid decline to stable adult dimensions by the end of adolescence.
15. The rate of metabolism
16. a
17. a. Hypoglycemia
    b. Elevated bilirubin levels
    c. Metabolic acidosis
18. 90
19. a. The difficult child
    b. The slow-to-warm-up child
    c. The easy child
20. behavior problems
21. a. 2
    b. 1
    c. 3
    d. 4
    e. 5
22. a. Trust vs. mistrust
    b. Autonomy vs. shame and doubt
    c. Initiative vs. guilt
    d. Industry vs. inferiority
    e. Identity vs. role confusion
23. a. 3, 5
    b. 1, 8
    c. 4, 7
    d. 2, 6

24. a
25. comprehension, expressed
26. a. Children conform to rules imposed by authority figures and are culturally oriented to the labels of good-bad and right-wrong.
    b. Children endeavor to define moral values and principles that the entire society agrees to. Emphasis is on the possibility of changing law in terms of societal needs.
    c. Children are concerned with conformity and loyalty, and with actively maintaining, supporting, and justifying the social order.
27. How the individual describes him or herself
28. a
29. b
30. Self-esteem
31. a. 2
    b. 5
    c. 1
    d. 4
    e. 3
32. a. Sensorimotor development
    b. Intellectual development
    c. Creativity
    d. Socialization
    e. Self-awareness
    f. Therapeutic value
    g. Moral value
33. parent-child
34. Denver-II
35. c
36. mothering person
37. c
38. d

Applying Critical Thinking to the Nursing Practice

A.
1. Yes
2. No, it does not. At 2 years of age, a child's height is typically 50% of his or her eventual adult height.
3. His mother demonstrates an appropriate response to him.

B.
1. It is important for health care providers to understand general patterns of development before performing an assessment of a child's developmental status.
2. a. Trust vs. mistrust: Trust develops when the child's

basic needs are consistently met. A specific intervention is to provide loving care. The unfavorable conflict is mistrust.
   b. Autonomy vs. shame and doubt: Autonomy allows the child to make choices. An intervention would be to give the child a sense of control over his or her environment by letting the child assist with the care routine. The unfavorable conflict is shame and doubt, which arises when children are made to feel small and self-conscious, when their choices are disastrous, when others shame them, or when they are forced to be dependent in areas in which they are capable of assuming control.
   c. Initiative vs. guilt: Initiative encourages exploration of the environment and setting realistic limits. An intervention would be to let the child choose when his or her bath will be given (in the morning or the evening). The unfavorable conflict is guilt. Children sometimes undertake goals or activities that are in conflict with those of parents or others, and being made to feel that their activities or imaginings are bad produces a sense of guilt.
   d. Industry vs. inferiority: Industry encourages competition, cooperation, and assisting in setting achievable goals. An intervention would be to have the child complete a task after setting a goal (eg, to learn how to keep his dressing clean and dry). The unfavorable conflict is inferiority, which may develop if too much is expected of children or if they believe that they cannot measure up to the standards set for them by others.
   e. Identity vs. role confusion: Identity provides positive feedback regarding appearance and activities. An intervention would be to provide

privacy for the adolescent to have some time alone while hospitalized. The unfavorable conflict is role confusion or the inability to establish new and separate roles, which will allow the child to enter the next stage of life.

3. a. No concept of right or wrong, no beliefs, and no convictions to guide behavior
   b. Imitation of religious gestures and behaviors of others without comprehension of meaning; typically, assimilation of some of the parents' values and beliefs
   c. Imitation of religious behavior and following of parental religious beliefs as part of daily lives without a real understanding of basic concepts
   d. Strong interest in religion with acceptance of a deity; making petitions to this deity and expecting them to be answered; a developing conscience that bothers them when they disobey; a reverence for thoughts and an ability to articulate their faith, perhaps even question its validity
   e. Realization that prayers are not always answered; initiation and then modification or abandonment of religious practices of their parents; beginning to determine which religious practices they will adopt and incorporate into their own set of values; perhaps comparing religious standards with a scientific viewpoint

C.

1. Any child can experience problems if there is incongruency between his or her temperament and the environment. Infants with difficult or slow-to-warm-up patterns of behavior are more vulnerable to the development of behavioral problems in early and middle childhood. Children of parents who fail to accept and connect with the child's temperamental behaviors often demonstrate behavioral problems.
2. a. Even-tempered, regular, predictable, adaptable, and open

   b. Highly active; irritable; irregular in habits; has negative withdrawal responses; slow to adapt to new routines, people, or situations

CHAPTER 4

Review of Essential Concepts

1. a. Privacy
   b. Minimal distractions
   c. Play opportunities for children while parent is interviewed
2. b
3. a
4. a
5. c
6. b
7. Any three of the following are acceptable:
   - Long periods of silence
   - Wide eyes and fixed facial expression
   - Constant fidgeting or attempting to move away
   - Nervous habits (eg, tapping)
   - Sudden disruptions
   - Looking around
   - Yawning
   - Frequently looking at a watch or clock
   - Attempting to change the topic of discussion
8. d
9. a. F
   b. T
   c. T
   d. T
10. a. 2
    b. 1
    c. 3
    d. 4
11. b.
12. Play
13. d
14. chief complaint
15. a
16. d
17. a
18. a. Approximate weight at 6 months, 1 year, 2 years, and 5 years of age
    b. Approximate length at 1 and 4 years of age
    c. Dentition, including age of onset, number of teeth, and symptoms during teething
19. a. The history uncovers areas of concern related to sexual activity.

   b. It alerts the nurse to circumstances that may indicate screening for sexually transmitted diseases or testing for pregnancy.
   c. It provides information related to the need for sexual counseling, such as safe sex practices.
20. b
21. b
22. "How has your child's general health been?" or "Has your child had any problems with his eyes, ears, nose, mouth, etc.?"
23. a. 3
    b. 1
    c. 2
    d. 4
24. a
25. Anthropometry
26. a. Malnourished
    b. At risk for becoming malnourished
    c. Well-nourished with adequate reserves
27. a
28. physical growth parameters
29. BMI (body mass index)-for-age
30. Nurses are often responsible for measuring growth in children.
31. d
32. length, height
33. Place your hand lightly above the infant's body to prevent accidental falls off the scale.
34. skinfold thickness
35. 36
36. respirations, pulse, temperature
37. 37° C to 37.5° C (98.6° F to 99.5° F)
38. Proper technique
39. Apical, Radial
40. Diaphragmatic
41. Appropriate cuff size
42. Any five of the following: hypovolemia, which may be induced by medications such as diuretics; vasodilation medications; prolonged immobility; dehydration; diarrhea; emesis; fluid loss from sweating and exertion; alcohol intake; dysrhythmias; diabetes mellitus; sepsis; and hemorrhage
43. 1 full minute
44. apically
45. a. 2
    b. 3
    c. 4
    d. 1

257

46. a. Inspection
    b. Palpation
47. a
48. Palpate nodes using the distal portion of the fingers and gently but firmly pressing in a circular motion along the regions where nodes are normally present.
49. d
50. PERRLA, which stands for pupils equal, round, react to light, and accommodation
51. a. Showing the child the instrument
    b. Demonstrating the light source and how it shines in the eye
    c. Explaining the reason for darkening the room
52. Snellen
53. renal anomalies, mental retardation
54. down, back; up, back
55. A translucent, light pearly pink or gray
56. Children often get upset with having to open their mouth.
57. b
58. a. Vesicular
    b. Bronchovesicular
    c. Bronchial
59. crackles, wheezes
60. younger than 7, older than 7
61. S1
62. a. Quality (They should be clear and distinct, not muffled, diffuse, or distant.)
    b. Intensity, especially in relation to the location or auscultatory site (They should not be weak or pounding.)
    c. Rate (They should have the same rate as the radial pulse.)
    d. Rhythm (They should be regular and even.)
63. a. Location of the area of the heart in which the murmur is heard best
    b. Time of the occurrence of the murmur within the S1–S2 cycle
    c. Intensity (evaluation in relationship to the child's position)
    d. Loudness
64. a. F. Palpation should be performed last so bowel sounds are not altered.
    b. T
    c. F. A femoral hernia occurs more often in girls.
    d. T

65. The best approach is to examine the genitalia matter-of-factly, placing no more emphasis on this part of the assessment than on any other segment. With an adolescent, this part of the assessment should be performed last. With both children and adolescents, privacy, respect, comfort, and confidentiality should be provided.
66. scoliosis
67. Pigeon toe, or toeing in, which usually results from torsional deformities, such as internal tibial torsion
68. push, pull
69. neurologic
70. tensing

Applying Critical Thinking to the Nursing Practice

A.

1. Introduce yourself to, and ask the name of, each family member who is present. Communicate with them using their preferred names, rather than using first names or "mother" or "father." Include children in the interaction by asking them their name, age, and other information.
2. It is important to include the parents in the problem-solving process because family-centered care is a holistic approach to nursing care that helps ensure the care plan is understood, implemented, and evaluated by the parent(s) and child working as a team.
3. One way is to use open-ended or broad questions, followed by guiding statements.
4. A number of techniques are effective. These include "I" messages, third-person technique, facilitative responding, storytelling, books, dreams, "what if" questions, three wishes, rating games, word association games, sentence completion, pros and cons, writing, drawing, magic, and play.

B.

1. Any four of the following are acceptable:
   - Learn proper terms of address.
   - Use a positive tone of voice to convey interest.

- Speak slowly and carefully, not loudly.
- Encourage questions.
- Learn basic words and sentences of the family's language.
- Avoid professional terms.
- Explain why questions are being asked.
- Repeat important information as needed.
- Explain in simple terms the reason or purpose for a treatment.
- Provide handouts written in the family's primary language.
- Make arrangements for an interpreter when necessary.
- Study about various cultures and learn from families and representatives of their culture.
- Use various methods of communicating information.
- Be sincere, open, and honest.

2. Tell the mother she can talk about the other children later in the interview. Then, at the end of the interview, allow her to verbalize her concerns and to ask basic questions.
3. He may not have received the immunizations required by law here in the United States; therefore it is important for the nurse to get a detailed history and accurate record of his immunizations from Mrs. Gonzales.
4. The nurse should obtain information concerning the age of Mrs. Gonzales and the father of Val, her marital status, and the current state of health and presence of existing illness of both parents. It is also important to know whether there is any evidence of heart disease, diabetes, stroke, high cholesterol, and similar conditions among first-degree relatives.

C.

1. a. 24-hour recall
   b. Food diary
   c. Food frequency record
2. Anthropometry is the measurement of height, weight, head circumference, proportions, skinfold thickness, and arm circumference. Skinfold thickness is a measurement of the body's

258

Answer Key

fat content and would be useful in determining whether Todd is overweight or obese.

3. a. Altered Nutrition: More Than Body Requirements related to eating practices
   b. Altered Nutrition: More Than Body Requirements related to knowledge deficit of parents

D.

1. Position the child comfortably in the mother's lap, with the child's knees flexed.

   Warm hands before touching skin.

   Use distraction.

   Teach the child to use deep breathing and to concentrate on an object.

   Begin with light and then move to deeper palpation.

   Palpate the most tender areas last.

   Have the child hold the parent's hand and squeeze if painful.

   Use the nonpalpating hand to comfort the child.

2. Have the child "help" by placing her hand over the nurse's hand.

   Have the child place her hand on her abdomen with fingers spread out wide. The nurse can then palpate between the child's fingers.

CHAPTER 5

Review of Essential Concepts

1. a
2. Behavioral assessment
3. For short, sharp procedural pain, such as during injections or lumbar punctures
4. Physiologic measures are not able to distinguish between physical responses to pain and other forms of stress to the body.
5. c
6. a
7. a
8. d
9. a
10. b
11. c
12. Oucher Pain Scale
13. To develop a trusting relationship with the child and the family, so that a deeper understanding of the pain experience may be obtained

14. Any four of the following are appropriate:
    - Distraction
    - Relaxation
    - Guided imagery
    - Positive self-talk
    - Thought stopping
    - Behavioral contracting
15. d
16. a. An increased frequency in quiet sleep
    b. Longer duration of quiet sleep
    c. Decreased crying in the neonatal intensive care unit
    d. Pain scores were significantly lower in kangaroo-held infants
17. a. Foods, special diets, herbal or plant preparations, vitamins, other supplements
    b. Chiropractic, osteopathy, massage
    c. Reiki, bioelectric or magnetic treatments, pulsed fields, alternating and direct currents
    d. Mental healing, expressive treatments, spiritual healing, hypnosis, relaxation
    e. Homeopathy; naturopathy; ayurvedic; and traditional Chinese medicine, which includes acupuncture and moxibustion
18. Nonopioids, including acetaminophen (Tylenol, paracetamol) and nonsteroidal antiinflammatory drugs (NSAIDs)
19. Opioids
20. d
21. Morphine
22. a. 3
    b. 2
    c. 1
    d. 5
    e. 4
    f. 8
    g. 6
    h. 7
23. When the analgesic controls pain without causing severe side effects in the patient
24. a. F. They metabolize more rapidly.
    b. T
    c. T
25. A ceiling effect means that dosages higher than the recommended dosage will not produce greater pain relief. A major difference between opioids and nonopioids is that nonopioids have a ceiling effect.

26. Children who are physically able to "push a button" (ie, 5 to 6 years of age) and who can understand the concept of pushing a button to obtain pain relief can use patient-controlled anesthesia.
27. d
28. Morphine
29. a. Patient controlled
    b. Nurse controlled
    c. Continuous basal rate infusion
30. a. 3
    b. 2
    c. 1
31. c
32. a. T
    b. F. They should not exceed the expected duration.
    c. F. It is not always appropriate, since not all pain is continuous.
    d. T
    e. T
    f. T
33. c
34. a. Tolerance
    b. Physical dependence
35. a. Irritability, tremors, seizures, increased motor tone, insomnia
    b. Nausea, vomiting, diarrhea, abdominal cramps
    c. Sweating, fever, chills, tachypnea, nasal congestion, rhinitis
36. b
37. Tolerance
38. Infants and children do not have the cognitive ability to make the cause-effect association and therefore cannot become addicted.
39. Pain relief scales or periodic ratings of pain intensity
40. b
41. a
42. a. 2
    b. 1
    c. 4
    d. 3
    e. 5
43. a. Increased heart rate
    b. Peripheral resistance
    c. Blood pressure
    d. Cardiac output
44. d
45. Severe pain
46. c
47. a. Teaching patients self-control skills to prevent headache (eg, biofeedback techniques, relaxation training)

b. Modifying behavior patterns that increase the risk of headache occurrence or that reinforce headache activity (eg, cognitive-behavioral stress management techniques)

48. Recurrent abdominal pain in children is pain that occurs at least once per month for three consecutive months, is accompanied by pain-free periods, and is severe enough that it interferes with a child's normal activities.

49. cognitive-behavioral

50. chronic pain

51. b

52. Painful peripheral neuropathy

53. a

54. To reduce the possibility that a child might experience unrelieved pain but be too sedated to report it

Applying Critical Thinking to the Nursing Practice

A.

1. You should notice Valery's facial expression (F), leg movement (L), activity (A), cry (C), and consolability (C). This tool measures pain by quantifying pain behaviors with scores ranging from 0 (no pain behaviors) to 10 (most possible pain behaviors). The Parent's Postoperative Pain Rating Scale could also be used.

2. It could be a combination of the following: heart rate, respiratory rate, blood pressure, palmar sweating, cortisone levels, transcutaneous oxygen, vagal tone, and endorphin concentrations. These reflect a generalized and complex response to stress.

3. The combination provides increased analgesia without increased side effects.

4. An antianxiety medication such as diazepam (Valium) or midazolam (Versed)

B.

1. Obtaining his level of pain by assessing his behaviors and placing these behaviors on a pain scale from 1 to 10

2. Pulmonary complications (pneumonia atelectasis) can occur after abdominal surgery and would affect his airway and breathing.

3. Acute pain can cause decreased muscle movement in the thorax and abdominal area, which leads to decreased tidal volume, vital capacity, functional residual capacity, and alveolar ventilation. If he is unable to cough and clear secretions because of his pain, the risk for complications such as pneumonia and atelectasis is high.

4. Pain related to surgical procedure

C.

You may see all the behaviors of a young child but less in the anticipatory stage. You might also see stalling behavior, such as "wait a minute" or "I need a minute first." Another expected finding is muscular rigidity, clenched fists, white knuckles, gritted teeth, contracted limbs, body stiffness, closed eyes, and wrinkled forehead.

D.

Administering nonopioid analgesics and placing the patient in the supine position for 1 hour after the procedure

CHAPTER 6

Review of Essential Concepts

1. b
2. c
3. a. 4
   b. 1
   c. 3
   d. 2
4. d
5. a
6. c
7. b
8. d
9. a
10. d
11. a
12. c
13. b
14. c
15. a
16. d
17. c
18. c
19. c
20. b
21. b
22. d
23. a
24. b
25. d
26. a
27. b
28. a
29. b
30. c
31. c
32. a
33. Intestinal parasitic diseases
34. b
35. a
36. b
37. d
38. Enterobiasis (pinworms)
39. pinworms
40. By performing a tape test
41. d
42. c
43. d
44. Scabies
45. Pediculosis capitis (head lice)
46. a

Applying Critical Thinking to the Nursing Practice

A.

1. Lyme disease

2. Laboratory diagnosis is completed with a two-step process including the screening test enzyme immunoassay or immunofluorescent immunoassay.

3. With oral doxycycline

4. Educating the parents to protect their children from exposure to ticks

B.

1. Axillary epitrochlear, cervical, submandibular, inguinal, and preauricular

2. Encephalitis, hepatitis, and Parinaud oculoglandular syndrome

3. History of contact with a cat or kitten, presence of regional lymphadenopathy for several days, and serologic identification of the causative organism by indirect fluorescent antibody assay or polymerase chain reaction test

CHAPTER 7

Review of Essential Concepts

1. a. T
   b. F. It is onset of breathing.
   c. T
   d. F. It decreases in pressure.
2. a
3. c

4. Newborns are predisposed to loss of body heat due to large surface area, little subcutaneous fat, and inability to shiver.
5. b
6. a
7. d
8. b
9. milia
10. a. Skin and mucous membranes
    b. Macrophage system
    c. Formation of antibodies to an antigen
11. c
12. a. F. The fovea centralis is not completely differentiated from the macula in the newborn.
    b. T
    c. T
    d. F. The newborn has the ability to distinguish among tastes and various types of solutions elicit differing facial reflexes
    e. T
13. a. Heart rate
    b. Respiratory effort
    c. Muscle tone
    d. Reflex irritability
    e. Color
14. c
15. Birth weight, gestational age
16. a. F. It is 13 to 14 inches.
    b. T
    c. F. The neonate loses about 10% of birth weight.
    d. F
    e. T
    f. T
17. a
18. b
19. d
20. Strabismus
21. The rooting reflex is elicited by stroking the cheek and noting the infant's response of turning toward the stimulated side and sucking.
22. The findings should be reported for further investigation.
23. c
24. Pseudomenstruation
25. a
26. b
27. A degree of paralysis from brain damage or nerve damage
28. b
29. a
30. An effective method of systematically assessing the infant's behavior

31. c
32. a. En face position
    b. Kissing, smiling
    c. Talking, cradling
    d. Holding, rocking
33. d
34. a. Tachypnea
    b. Nasal flaring
    c. Grunting
    d. Intercostal retractions
    e. Cyanosis
35. a. Evaporation
    b. Radiation
    c. Conduction
    d. Convection
36. hand washing
37. c
38. The typical abductor is a female between the ages of 12 and 55 who is often overweight and has low self-esteem; she may be emotionally disturbed because of the loss of her own child or an inability to conceive and may have a strained relationship with her husband or partner.
39. d
40. To prevent hemorrhagic disease of the newborn
41. To educate parents regarding the importance of screening and to collect appropriate specimens at the recommended time (after 24 hours of age)
42. The uppermost horny layer of the epidermis; sweat; superficial fat; metabolic products; and external substances, such as amniotic fluid, microorganisms, and chemicals
43. 5, 15
44. a. F. Infants can feel pain.
    b. T
45. Breast milk consists of a number of bioavailable micronutrients, meaning these nutrients are available in quantities and qualities that make them easily digestible by the newborn's intestine and absorbed for energy and growth.
46. a. Respiratory infections
    b. Gastrointestinal infections
    c. Numerous allergies
    d. Type 2 diabetes
    e. Atopy
47. a. Early separation of mother and newborn
    b. Delays in initiating breastfeeding
    c. Provision of formula in the hospital and in discharge packs

    d. Conflicting information by health care workers
    e. Formula coupons given at discharge
48. The American Academy of Pediatrics recommends breastfeeding until at least 1 year of age as the best form of infant nutrition.
49. Desire to breastfeed, satisfaction with breastfeeding, and available support systems
50. a. Absence of a rigid feeding schedule
    b. Correct positioning of the infant at the breast to achieve latch-on
    c. Correct sucking technique
51. Hold them close to the body while rocking or cuddling them.
52. c
53. a. Cow's milk–based formulas
    b. Soy milk–based formulas
    c. Whey-hydrolysate formulas
    d. Amino acid formulas
54. b
55. a. Recognizing individual differences and explaining to parents that such characteristics are normal
    b. Enhancing the infant's development during awake periods
56. c
57. a. Pointing out normal characteristics
    b. Encouraging identification through consistent referral to the child by name
    c. Encouraging the father to cuddle, hold, talk to, or feed the infant
    d. Demonstrating, whenever necessary, the soothing powers of caressing, stroking, and rocking the child
58. Recognizing the individuality of the children
59. Before birth
60. Postpartum hospitalizations are shorter.
61. 1 year

Applying Critical Thinking to the Nursing Practice

A.
1. fewer than 100 beats/min
2. Any of the following are acceptable:
   • The degree of physiologic immaturity

261

- Infection
- Congenital malformations
- Maternal sedation or analgesia
- Neuromuscular disorders
3. He is in the first period of reactivity.
4. c

B.
1. Perinatal mortality and morbidity are related to gestational age.
2. a. Posture
   b. Square window
   c. Arm recoil
   d. Popliteal angle
   e. Scarf sign
   f. Heel-to-ear maneuver
3. his or her weight falls between the 10th and 90th percentiles

C.
1. meconium; It is composed of amniotic fluid and its constituents, intestinal secretions, shed mucosal cells, and possibly blood (ingested maternal blood or minor bleeding of alimentary tract vessels).
2. It usually appears by the third day after initiation of feeding; is greenish brown to yellowish brown, thin, and less sticky than meconium; and may contain some milk curds.
3. In breastfed infants, stools are yellow to golden, are pasty in consistency, and have an odor similar to that of sour milk. In formula-fed infants, stools are pale yellow to light brown, are firmer in consistency, and have a more offensive odor.

D.
1. Microcephaly or craniostenosis
2. The absence of arm movement signals a potential birth injury paralysis, such as Klumpke or Erb-Duchenne palsy.

E.
1. Any three of the following are acceptable:
   - Ineffective Airway Clearance related to excess mucus, improper positioning
   - Risk for Altered Body Temperature related to immature temperature control or change in environmental temperature
   - Risk for Infection related to deficient immunologic defenses, environmental factors, or maternal disease

- Risk for Trauma related to physical helplessness
- Altered Nutrition: Less Than Body Requirements (potential), related to immaturity or parental knowledge deficit
- Altered Family Processes related to maturational crisis, birth of full-term infant, or change in family unit

2. Any four of the following are acceptable:
   - Suction the mouth and nasopharynx with a bulb syringe.
   - Position the infant on his right side after feeding.
   - Position the infant on his back during sleep.
   - Perform as few procedures as possible on the infant during the first hour of life.
   - Take vital signs.
   - Observe for signs of respiratory distress.
   - Keep diapers, clothing, and blankets loose.
   - Clean nares of crusted material.
   - Check for patency of nares.
   - Keep the head of the bed elevated.
3. The airway remains patent, breathing is regular and unlabored, and the infant has a normal respiratory rate.
4. The parents should be instructed on routine baby care such as feeding, bathing, and umbilical and circumcision care. They should also be encouraged to participate in parenting classes, and the use of car restraints should be discussed.

CHAPTER 8

Review of Essential Concepts

1. c.
2. a
3. fractured clavicle
4. Pressure on the facial nerve (cranial nerve VII) during delivery, causing facial nerve paralysis
5. a. 2
   b. 3
   c. 1
6. a. 4
   b. 3
   c. 2
   d. 1

7. high-risk newborn
8. By birth weight, gestational age, and predominant pathophysiologic problems
9. apical heart rate
10. a
11. c
12. neutral thermal environment
13. a. Hypoxia
    b. Metabolic acidosis
    c. Hypoglycemia
14. a. Daily (at least) weighs
    b. Accurate intake and output of all fluids, including medications and blood products
15. c
16. c
17. c
18. donor milk
19. weight gain, tolerance
20. b
21. a
22. a. A strong, vigorous suck
    b. Coordination of sucking and swallowing
    c. A gag reflex
    d. Sucking on the gavage tube, hands, or a pacifier
    e. Rooting and wakefulness before and after feedings
23. prone
24. c
25. d
26. d
27. c
28. Any two of the following would be acceptable:
    - Closing doors (eg, incubator portholes)
    - Not listening to loud radios or talking loudly
    - Not handling noisy equipment (eg, trash containers)
29. Any two of the following would be acceptable:
    - Darkening the room
    - Covering the crib
    - Placing eye patches over the infant's eyes at night
30. a
31. b
32. c
33. a
34. a. 1
    b. 3
    c. 2
35. c
36. d
37. a
38. d

39. O, A, B
40. Exchange transfusion
41. c
42. a. Provide adequate oxygen to the tissues
    b. Prevent lactic acid accumulation resulting from hypoxia
    c. Avoid the potentially negative effects of oxygen and barotrauma
43. b
44. c
45. d
46. Jitteriness is not accompanied by ocular movement, whereas seizures are. Whereas the dominant movement in jitteriness is tremor, seizure movement is clonic jerking that cannot be stopped by flexion of the affected limb. Jitteriness is highly sensitive to stimulation, but seizures are not.
47. c
48. b
49. b
50. An acute inflammatory disease of the bowel that has increased incidence in preterm infants
51. a. Intestinal ischemia
    b. Colonization by pathogenic bacteria
    c. Substrate in intestine
52. Any four or more of the following would be acceptable:
    • Abdominal distention
    • Blood in stools or gastric contents
    • Gastric retention
    • Localized abdominal wall erythema or induration
    • Bilious vomiting
    • Lethargy
    • Apnea
    • Poor feeding
    • Decreased urinary output
    • Unstable temperature
53. euglycemic
54. b
55. d
56. a
57. c
58. b
59. d
60. Toxoplasmosis, other, rubella, cytomegalovirus infection, herpes simplex
61. teratogen; alcohol, tobacco, antiepileptics, isotretinoin, lithium, cocaine, diethylstilbestrol
62. b
63. a
64. Galactosemia

Applying Critical Thinking to the Nursing Practice

A.

1. a. Caput succedaneum is a vaguely outlined area of edematous tissue situated over the portion of the scalp that presents in a vertex delivery. The swelling consists of serum, blood, or both, accumulated in the tissues above the bone, and it may extend beyond the bone margins. It is present within 24 hours of birth. The injury usually disappears after a few days.
   b. Cephalhematoma is formed when blood vessels rupture during labor or delivery, producing bleeding into the area between the bone and its periosteum. The boundaries are sharply demarcated and do not extend beyond the limits of the bone. Swelling is usually minimal at birth and increases on the second or third day. It is absorbed within 2 weeks to 3 months.

2. Early signs of subgaleal hemorrhage are detected through serial head circumference measurements and inspection of the back of the neck for increasing edema. Subgaleal hemorrhage is indicated by a firm mass or a boggy fluctuant mass over the scalp that crosses the suture line and moves as the baby is repositioned. Other signs include pallor, tachycardia, increasing head circumference, and forward and lateral positioning of the newborn's ears because the hematoma extends posteriorly.

B.

1. The nurse considers the individual infant's readiness, rather than initiating feedings based on weight and age or a predetermined time schedule. Feeding readiness is determined by each infant's medical status, energy level, ability to sustain a brief quiet alert state, gag reflex (demonstrated with a gavage tube insertion), spontaneous rooting and sucking behaviors, and functional sucking reflex.

2. Disturbing the infant as little as possible, maintaining a neutral thermal environment, gavage feeding as appropriate, promoting oxygenation, judiciously implementing any caregiving activities that increase oxygen and caloric consumption

3. Prone position is best for most preterm infants and results in improved oxygenation, better-tolerated feedings, and more organized sleep-rest patterns. Infants exhibit less physical activity and energy expenditure when placed in the prone position. Prolonged supine positioning for preterm infants is not desirable, because they appear to lose their sense of equilibrium when supine and use vital energy in attempts to recover balance by postural changes. In addition, prolonged supine positioning is associated with long-term problems, such as decreased flexion of the limbs, pelvis, and trunk; widely abducted hips (frog-leg position); retracted and abducted shoulders; ankle and foot eversion; increased neck extension; and increased trunk extension with neck and back arching. When medically stable, preterm infants should also be placed in a supine position to sleep, unless conditions such as gastroesophageal reflux or upper airway anomalies make this impractical. Prone positioning for play should be provided in the nursery. Before discharge, the nurse should demonstrate for the parents how to position the infant supine, how to provide comfort such as a pacifier during the transition from prone to supine, and how to use neck rolls to make the position more comfortable for the infant, where the limbs and trunk are in flexion and the infant's hands are to his or her face at midline.

4. Any four of the following answers are correct:
   • Clustering care so that the family can have quality time bonding with the infant

- Turning down the lights
- Assessing for signs of appropriate stimulation
- When signs of overstimulation are observed, implementing interventions to decrease this stimulation
- Providing a comforting touch
- Adequately managing the infant's pain
- Providing stimulating sights, smells, and sounds for the infant
- Offering stimulus during periods of alertness
- Keeping interventions as short as possible
- Providing times of uninterrupted sleep
- Beginning one type of stimulus at a time
- Providing firm boundaries (nesting)
- Encouraging kangaroo care
- Reducing noise levels
- Having the mother softly speak to her infant or playing tapes of the parents' and siblings' voices
- Positioning with limbs and trunk in flexion and hands to face at midline
- Avoiding quick position changes
- Dipping pacifiers in mother's breast milk for nonnutritive sucking
- Initiating eye contact as appropriate for the infant's level of stimulation

C.
1. a. Immaturity of hepatic function
   b. Increased bilirubin load from increased hemolysis of red blood cells
2. a. After 24 hours
   b. By the third day
   c. By the fifth day
3. a. Shield the infant's eyes with an opaque mask.
   b. Place the infant nude under the fluorescent light with a Plexiglas shield.
   c. Monitor body temperature.
   d. Give additional fluids.
   e. Provide meticulous skin care.
4. a. Parental anxiety
   b. Less eye-to-eye contact because of eye patches
   c. Interruption of breastfeeding for phototherapy

D.
1. Nosocomially through cross-contamination; the sources of this could include a humidifying apparatus, suction machines, improper use of sterile technique, inadequate education and performance of handwashing skills, or indwelling catheters and the like.
2. Some of the signs of sepsis are poor temperature control, pallor, hypotension, edema, respiratory distress, diminished or increased activity, full fontanel, poor feeding, vomiting, diarrhea, jaundice, and an infant not doing well.
3. Identification of the existing problem

E.
1. Hypoglycemia is common and occurs as a result of the hyperplasia and hypertrophy of the islet cells in utero. The islet cells continue to excrete large amounts of insulin after birth, resulting in decreased blood glucose levels (hypoglycemia).
2. They help prevent hypoglycemia.
3. a. Brachial plexus injury and palsy
   b. Fractured clavicle
   c. Phrenic nerve palsy

CHAPTER 9

Review of Essential Concepts

1. John's weight will double in the first 6 months, and he should grow approximately 2.5 cm per month. His weight should be approximately 7 kg (15.5 pounds), and his height should be approximately 66 cm (25.9 inches).
2. a. The close proximity of the trachea to the bronchi
   b. The short, straight eustachian tube closely communicates with the ear
   c. The inability of the immune system to produce immunoglobulin A (IgA)
3. 6 months of age
4. The liver
5. a. Greater proportion of extracellular fluid
   b. Immaturity of renal structures
6. At 1 month of age, the hands are predominately closed, and at 3 months of age, they are predominately open.
7. d
8. 4 to 6 months
9. The quality of both the parent (caregiver)–child relationship and the care the infant receives
10. Sensorimotor
11. a. Separation
    b. Achievement of the concept of object permanence
    c. Ability to use symbols or mental representation
12. Reactive attachment disorder
13. 4 to 8 months
14. Crying
15. 10 to 11 months
16. a. Interpersonal contact
    b. Recreational and educational stimulation
17. a. T
    b. T
    c. F
    d. T
    e. T
18. Iron
19. 5
20. After 1 year of age
21. Infant cereal is introduced because of its high iron content.
22. a. Disappearance of the extrusion reflex and swallowing is more coordinated
    b. Head control is well developed
    c. Voluntary grasping and improved eye-hand coordination
    d. Maturation of the gastrointestinal tract
23. a. T
    b. F. All infants should receive a daily supplement of vitamin D until the infant is consuming at least 1 L/day of vitamin D–fortified formula.
    c. F. Some infants may have drooling, increased finger sucking, or biting hard objects but fever, vomiting, or diarrhea are not common symptoms and warrant further investigation.
    d. F. Iron should not be administered with whole cow's milk or milk products because it binds free iron and prevents absorption; iron supplements should be administered between meals for greater absorption.

24. 4 to 7 days
25. a. Suffocation
    b. Motor vehicle–related death
    c. Drowning
26. Fall-related injuries
27. back

Applying Critical Thinking to the Nursing Practice

A.

1. a. Differential crying, smiling, and vocalization (more to the mother than anyone else)
   b. Visual-motor orientation (looking more at the mother, even if she is not close)
   c. Crying when the mother leaves the room
   d. Approaching through location (crawling, creeping, or walking)
   e. Clinging (especially in the presence of a stranger)
2. Educate Tami about the need for other family members to provide close physical contact and consistent and loving care. Infants begin attaching to other members of the family about one month after showing attachment to the mother (or primary caregiver).

B.

1. a. Start Beverly on cereal first.
   b. Mix cereal with formula or breast milk.
   c. Introduce spoon feeding after Beverly has had some formula or breast milk.
   d. Beverly may at first push the spoon away; be persistent.
   e. Introduce new foods one at a time. New foods are fed in small amounts (about 1 teaspoon) for a period of 4 to 7 days.
   f. As the amount of solids increases, decrease the amount of formula.
   g. Do not introduce foods by mixing them with formula or breast milk in the bottle.
2. The nurse should explain that the majority of the infant's caloric needs is derived from the primary milk source (human or formula); therefore solids should not be perceived as a substitute for milk until Beverly is older than 12 months.

3. Parents can give the infant a cold teething ring but encourage them not to freeze the teething ring as the gels or non-sterile water may crack and leak into the infant's mouth; systematic analgesics (acetaminophen or ibuprofen) can be given if age appropriate for no more than 3 days; nonprescription topical anesthetic ointments should only be used under the advice and supervision of a health care provider.

C.

1. Such developmental landmarks include crawling, standing, cruising, walking, climbing, pulling on objects, throwing objects, picking up small objects, exploring by mouthing, and exploring away from the parent.
2. a. Place guards around heating appliances, fireplaces, or furnaces.
   b. Keep electrical wires hidden or out of reach.
   c. Place plastic guards or caps over electrical outlets; place furniture in front of outlets.
   d. Keep a hanging tablecloth out of reach.
   e. Smoke detectors should be tested and operating properly.
   f. Check the temperature of food after warming it up.
   g. Lower the water heater to a safe temperature.
   h. Turn handles of cooking utensils toward the back of the stove.
   i. Have the child wear flame-retardant fabric.
   j. All small appliances, such as an iron, should be turned off, disconnected, and placed out of reach when not in use.
3. Infants at this age still explore objects by mouthing them and might choke on a small object.
4. The child may get into the purse or handbag because of their curiosity, ingest the medication, and accidentally be poisoned.
5. Place a fence around the swimming pool with a gate lock that is out of any child's reach; supervise the infant in the water at all times; swimming lessons are encouraged but are not foolproof for preventing drowning.

CHAPTER 10

Review of Essential Concepts

1. a. Children exclusively breast-fed by mothers who have an inadequate intake of vitamin D or children who are exclusively breastfed longer than 6 months without adequate maternal vitamin D intake or supplementation
   b. Children with dark skin pigmentation who are exposed to minimal sunlight because of socioeconomic, religious, or cultural beliefs; housing in urban areas of high pollution; or live above or below a latitude of 33 degrees north and south
   c. Children with diets that are low in sources of vitamin D and calcium
   d. Individuals who use milk products not supplemented with vitamin D (eg, yogurt, raw cow's milk) as the primary source of milk
   e. Children who are overweight or obese
2. 10 times
3. Folic acid, 0.4 mg/day
4. Nutritional failure to thrive
5. Whole cow's milk
6. Salicylates
7. fat-soluble
8. Vitamin B12
9. a. Lack of food (inadequate food intake)
   b. Diarrhea (gastroenteritis)
10. Cystic fibrosis; cancer; chronic diarrhea syndromes; HIV; burns; inborn errors of metabolism; gastrointestinal malabsorption
11. Thin, wasted extremities and a prominent abdomen from edema
12. Marasmus
13. a. Rehydration with an oral rehydration solution that also replaces electrolytes
    b. Administration of antibiotics to prevent recurrent infections
    c. Provision of adequate nutrition by either breastfeeding or a proper weaning diet
14. 50
15. An acute asthma attack (wheezing, decreased air movement in airways, dyspnea)

16. a. Wear medical identification such as a bracelet.
    b. Have an injectable epinephrine cartridge (EpiPen) readily available and know how to use it.
    c. Have a copy of the individualized written treatment plan on hand for prompt diagnosis and treatment.
17. A double blind, placebo-controlled food challenge
18. Crying and fussing for more than 3 hours a day occurring more than 3 days per week and for more than 3 weeks in a healthy infant
19. a. Infant's diet
    b. Diet of the breastfeeding mother
    c. Time of day when crying occurs
    d. Relationship of crying to feeding times
    e. Presence of specific family members during crying and those family members' habits, such as smoking
    f. Activity of caregiver before, during, and after the crying
    g. Characteristics of the cry (duration, intensity)
    h. Measures used to relieve the crying and their effectiveness
    i. The infant's stooling, voiding, and sleep patterns
20. Reassuring both parents that they are not doing anything wrong and that the infant is not experiencing any physical or emotional harm
21. Through their assessment of the child, parents, and family interactions
22. Reversing the cause of the growth failure
23. Isolation, social crisis, inadequate support systems, poor parenting role models
24. Place the infant in a prone position
25. supine
26. Low birth weight or preterm birth; low Apgar scores; recent viral illness; siblings of two or more sudden infant death syndrome victims; male gender; American Indian or African-American ethnicity
27. Anything that suggests they are responsible for the infant's death
28. pacifier use

29. continuous recording of cardio-respiratory patterns (cardiopneumogram or pneumocardiogram)
30. The infant's clinical condition and when infants have gone 2 or 3 months without significant episodes requiring intervention
31. a. Removing leads from the infant when not attached to the monitor
    b. Unplugging the power cord from the electrical outlet when not plugged into the monitor
    c. Using safety covers on electrical outlets

Applying Critical Thinking to the Nursing Practice

A.
1. Food allergy, or hypersensitivity, is a reaction involving immunologic mechanisms, usually immunoglobulin E (IgE); the reactions may be immediate or delayed and mild or severe, such as anaphylactic reaction. Food intolerance, on the other hand, refers to reactions involving known or unknown nonimmunologic mechanisms; lactose intolerance is an example of a reaction that looks like allergy but is due to deficiency of the enzyme lactase.
2. Food allergy

B.
1. Loud crying spells lasting for 4 hours for the past 3 weeks, pulling his feet up toward his abdomen, and thriving normally despite the pain reaction
2. Changing the formula or eliminating cow's milk protein from breastfeeding mothers, and behavioral interventions (massage infant's abdomen, respond immediately to crying, swaddle infant, change environment, add a pacifier)

C.
1. Monitors can cause electrical burns and electrocution.
2. Inform the utility company so that if there is a power outage, emergency power may be provided. Notify the rescue squad so that if the infant stops breathing, they will be aware of the problem and may respond more quickly to a call.
3. used, response

CHAPTER 11

Review of Essential Concepts

1. Between 12 and 36 months
2. 2½ years
3. T
4. T
5. F. The respiratory and heart rate slows.
6. elimination
7. 18 and 24 months
8. a. Differentiation of self from others, particularly the mother
    b. Toleration of separation from the parent
    c. Ability to withstand delay gratification
    d. Control over bodily functions
    e. Acquisition of socially acceptable behavior
    f. Verbal means of communication
    g. Ability to interact with others in a less egocentric manner
9. Acquiring a sense of autonomy while overcoming doubt and shame
10. Negativism is an attempt by children to express their will by using words such as "no." This frequently disrupts the environment. On the other hand, ritualism is the need to maintain sameness and reliability, providing a sense of comfort in the environment.
11. ego
12. The final sensorimotor stage, invention of new means through mental combinations
13. In this stage, children cannot think in terms of operations—that is, the ability to manipulate objects in relation to each other in a logical fashion. Rather, toddlers think primarily on the basis of their perception of an event. Problem solving is based on what they see or hear directly, rather than on what they recall about objects and events.
14. Family and environment
15. 2 years
16. 3 years
17. a. The child's emergence from a symbiotic fusion with the mother
    b. Those achievements that mark a child's assumption of their individual characteristics in the environment
18. Rapprochement

19. 300, 65%
20. They can feed themselves, drink well from a covered cup, and manage a spoon with considerable spilling.
21. Toddlers engage in parallel play alongside, not with, other children. There is less emphasis on the exclusive use of one sensory modality. The toddler inspects the toy, talks to the toy, tests its strength and durability, and invents several uses for it. Imitation is one of the most distinguishing characteristics of play and enriches children's opportunity to engage in fantasy.
22. T
23. a. Waking up dry from a nap or overnight sleep
    b. Being aware of the urge to void or stool
    c. Communicating the need to go
    d. Being dry for at least 2 hours during the day
24. A good time to start talking about the new baby is when the toddler becomes aware of the pregnancy and of the changes taking place in the home in anticipation of the new member.
25. include
26. Consistency and developmentally appropriate expectations and rewards
27. By reducing the opportunities for a "no" answer
28. Physiologic anorexia
29. 1 tablespoon
30. Brushing and flossing
31. A "smear" or "rice-size" amount for children less than 3 years of age and a "pea-size" amount should be used in children 3 to 6 years of age
32. As soon as the bristles are frayed or bent
33. Motor vehicle injuries
34. Rearward facing
35. 8 to 12 years
36. Scald burns
37. Improper storage of toxic agents

Applying Critical Thinking to the Nursing Practice

A.
1. a. Falls at the 75th percentile
   b. Falls at the 75th percentile
2. The nurse needs to explain to the mother that growth slows during the toddler years. She would benefit from knowing that a toddler gains approximately 4 to 6 pounds and grows 3 inches per year.
3. a. Goes up and down stairs alone, using both feet on each step; runs fairly well, with a wide stance; picks up objects without falling; and can kick a ball forward without overbalancing
   b. Can build a tower of six or seven cubes; aligns two or more cubes like a train; turns the pages of a book one at a time; can imitate vertical and circular strokes when drawing; and turns doorknobs and unscrews lids
   c. Has a vocabulary of 300 words; uses two- or three-word phrases; uses the pronouns I, me, and you; understands directional commands; gives first name; verbalizes need for toileting; and talks incessantly
4. The nurse should let the mother know this is a normal characteristic of parallel play, which is typical during the toddler years.
5. a. Selection of appropriate toys must involve safety factors, especially in relation to size and sturdiness.
   b. Allow children to play with a variety of toys that foster creative thinking rather than passive toys that the child observes; the child should be allowed to choose the toys he wishes to play with at a given time.
6. b
7. a. When a child is routinely given a bottle of juice or milk at naptime or bedtime or uses the bottle as a pacifier while awake
   b. Frequent nocturnal breast-feeding for prolonged periods
   c. Coating pacifiers with honey
   d. Prolonged bottle feeding

B.
1. Toddlers give a persistent "no" response to most requests. Interventions include decreasing the opportunity for the word "no" by offering the toddler choices.
2. As an assertion of self-control and an attempt to control the environment, it increases independence. Interventions include educating the parents so they recognize that this is a normal and natural step in the toddler's development.
3. Toddlers assert their independence by violently objecting in this manner to restrictions on their behavior. Interventions include educating the parents to allow some independence with restrictions on the behalf of their toddler so he or she can progress and develop in a healthy way.
4. a. Are picky, fussy eaters with strong taste preferences
   b. Enjoy eating with their fingers and enjoy foods of different colors and shapes
   c. Like predictability and rituals involving mealtime and utensils
   d. Have unpredictable table manners
5. This is important because the eating habits established in early childhood tend to have lasting effects, such as the prevention of obesity and cardiovascular disease. Interventions include educating parents about healthy choices for toddlers and discussing the importance of role modeling healthy eating.
6. Daily stressors such as toilet training, moving, sibling birth, experiences of loss, or separation from parents
7. a. Provide a light snack
   b. Use of transitional objects
   c. Avoid stimulating activities and make the hour before bedtime a quiet time of reading

C.
1. a. One-on-one and face-to-face education
   b. Safety interventions and safety equipment
2. The toddler has found new freedom in his or her increased locomotion and is unaware of danger in the environment.
3. a. Motor vehicle injuries
   b. Drowning
   c. Burns
   d. Accidental poisoning
   e. Falls

267

Answer Key

f. Choking and suffocation
g. Bodily injury
4. Any five of the following are acceptable:
   - Matches and cigarette lighters
   - Sources of water—tubs, swimming pools
   - Medications, toxic agents, plants
   - Unguarded stairways
   - Uncovered electrical outlets
   - Tools, garden equipment
   - Firearms
5. a. 1, 3, 4, 5, 8, 9
   b. 1, 2, 4, 5, 6, 7
   c. 3, 8
   d. 2, 4, 5, 7

CHAPTER 12

Review of Essential Concepts

1. slows, stabilizes
2. F. Preschoolers are slender, sturdy, graceful, agile, and posturally erect
3. T
4. 5 years
5. Initiative; Guilt
6. a. Readiness for school
   b. Scholastic learning
7. a. The preconceptual phase (ages 2 to 4 years)
   b. The phase of intuitive thought (ages 4 to 7 years)
8. Play
9. T
10. Causality resembles logical thought. Preschoolers explain a concept as they have heard it described by others, but their understanding is limited. The concept of time is an example of causality.
11. Because of their egocentrism and transductive reasoning, preschoolers believe their thoughts are all-powerful.
12. T
13. conscience
14. T
15. Intrusive experiences are frightening, especially those that disrupt the integrity of the skin, such as injections and surgery. They fear that if their skin is "broken," all of their blood and "insides" can leak out. Therefore bandages are critical to "keep everything from coming out."
16. opposite-sex, same-sex

17. 2100 words
18. Children aged 3 to 4 years can speak in sentences of three or four words. Their speech is telegraphic. They ask questions and use plurals and past tense verbs. They can name familiar objects. Children aged 4 to 5 years use sentences of four to five words. They can repeat a question until they receive an answer.
19. Associative play is defined as group play in similar or identical activities but without rigid organization or rules.
20. a. They become friends for the child in times of loneliness.
    b. They accomplish what the child is still attempting.
    c. They experience what the child wants to forget or remember.
21. Social and emotional maturity, especially attention span and academic readiness
22. a. Learning group cooperation
    b. Adjusting to various socio-cultural differences
    c. Coping with frustration, dissatisfaction, and anger
23. Personal observation
24. a. Determine what the child knows and thinks.
    b. Be honest.
25. Masturbation
26. a. Fear of the dark
    b. Fear of being left alone
    c. Fear of animals
    d. Fear of ghosts
    e. Fear of sexual matters
    f. Fear of objects or persons associated with pain
27. By actively involving them in finding practical methods to deal with the frightening experience
28. Because of their limited capacity to cope
29. a. Quantity (number of occurrences)
    b. Severity (interference with social or cognitive function)
    c. Distribution (different manifestations)
    d. Onset (when behavior started)
    e. Duration (at least 4 weeks)
30. 2 and 4 years
31. Stuttering; Boys
32. T
33. 13 to 19 g/day
34. 5 servings

35. Fruit juices and other sugar-sweetened beverages
36. T
37. T
38. T

Applying Critical Thinking to the Nursing Practice

A.

1. a. Slightly above the 25th percentile
   b. Falls just below the 50th percentile
2. Physical growth of a preschooler slows and stabilizes. The average child gains about 2 to 3 kg (4.5 to 6.5 pounds) per year and increases in height by about 6.5 to 9 cm (2.5 to 3.5 inches) per year.
3. a. Skips and hops on alternate feet; throws and catches a ball well; jumps rope; skates with good balance; walks backward with heel to toe; jumps from a height of 12 inches and lands on his toes; balances on alternate feet with his eyes closed
   b. Ties shoelaces; uses scissors, simple tools, or pencil well; copies a diamond and triangle; adds seven to nine parts to stick figure; prints a few letters, numbers, or words
   c. Has a vocabulary of 2100 words; uses six- to eight-word sentences; names coins and names four or more colors; describes drawing; knows days of the week and names of months; can follow three commands in succession
4. The nurse could inform Thom's mother that imaginary friends typically show up at around 3 years of age and stop when the child enters school. Firstborn children are more likely to have an imaginary friend. It might help to inform Thom's mother that imaginary friends serve three purposes: they become friends in times of loneliness, they accomplish what the child is still attempting, and they experience what the child wants to forget or remember. Reassure Thom's mother that his fantasy is a sign of health that helps him differentiate between make-believe and reality.

268

Answer Key

5. a Jumping, running, climbing, swimming, skating, tricycles, wagons, gym and sports equipment, sandboxes, wading pools, and activities at water parks
   b. Dress-up clothes, dolls, housekeeping toys, dollhouses, play store toys, telephones, toy farm animals and equipment, village sets, trains, trucks, cars, planes, hand puppets, and medical kits
6. The nurse could inform Thom's mother to expect a tranquil period at 5 years of age; help Thom's mother prepare him for entrance into school; ensure he is up-to-date on immunizations; suggest that unemployed parental caregivers consider their own activities when Thom begins school; and suggest swimming lessons or other activities for Thom.

B.
1. The social climate, type of guidance, and attitude toward the children fostered by the teacher or leader rather than whether structured learning is imposed
2. a. Facility's daily program
   b. Teacher qualifications
   c. Staff-to-student ratio
   d. Discipline policy
   e. Environmental safety precautions
   f. Provision of meals
   g. Sanitary conditions
3. a. Present the idea of school as exciting and pleasurable.
   b. Talk to the child about the activities that he or she will participate in at school.
   c. Introduce the child to the teacher and familiarize him or her with the school.
   d. Provide the school with detailed information about the child's home environment, such as familiar routines, favorite activities, food preferences, and personal habits.

C.
1. At about age 3 years, children are aware of anatomic differences between the sexes and are concerned with how the anatomy of the opposite sex works. This leads to physical exploration and questions to obtain more information. In addition, preschoolers have been exposed to a large amount of information and are constantly searching for explanations.
2. Sleep disturbances are typically related to negative sleep associations, nighttime fears, inconsistent bedtime routines, and lack of limit setting. As toddlers and preschoolers cope with autonomy and separation, they have more sleep problems.
3. The frequency of professional dental care should be based on a child's individual risk assessment including family history, sociodemographic factors, the child's dental development, the presence or absence of dental disease, special health care needs, and dietary habits.
4. The American Academy of Pediatrics Committee on Nutrition recommends that total fat consumption should be 30% of caloric intake over several days. Parents should provide foods with less saturated fat (eg, low-fat milk).
5. Carbonated beverages are known to contribute to dental caries, and they also provide nonnutritive calories that may displace or preclude the intake of nutrients necessary for growth.

CHAPTER 13

Review of Essential Concepts

1. a. Daytime tiredness
   b. Behavior changes
   c. Hyperactivity
   d. Difficulty concentrating and impaired learning ability
   e. Poor control of emotions and impulses
   f. Strain on family relationships
2. Cultural
3. a. Evening media use
   b. Daytime exposure to violent media content
4. a. Provide a consistent bedtime ritual.
   b. Ignore attention-seeking behavior.
   c. The child should not be taken into the parents' bed or allowed to stay up past a reasonable hour.
5. Nightmares are scary dreams that take place during rapid eye movement (REM) sleep and are followed by full awakening. After the nightmare is over, the child wakes and cries. Night terrors are a partial arousal from very deep non-REM sleep. The child screams and thrashes during the terror and then is calm.
6. Contact dermatitis
7. To prevent further exposure of the skin to the offending substance
8. Oil and urushiol
9. The area should be immediately flushed with cold running water.
10. Scorpions, the brown recluse spider, the black widow spider
11. Saline or lactated Ringer
12. Puncture wounds or wounds in areas where infection could result in cosmetic (face) or functional impairment (hand)
13. prevention
14. Because human dental plaque and gingiva harbor pathogenic organisms, and delayed treatment increases the risk of infection
15. Toddlers
16. a. Percentage of total body surface area burned
    b. Depth of the burn
17. a. 2
    b. 1
    c. 3
    d. 4
18. F. A burn that is 10% of the total body surface area can be life threatening if not treated correctly.
19. Wheezing, increasing secretions, hoarseness, wet rales, and carbonaceous secretions; these manifestations may be delayed as long as 24 to 48 hours.
20. Airway compromise and profound burn shock
21. pulmonary edema
22. a. F. It is not helpful to place a wet dressing on a burn victim. Wet dressings promote vasoconstriction, which impairs circulation to the burned area and increases tissue damage.
    b. T
    c. T
    d. F. Burned clothing is removed to prevent further damage from smoldering fabric and hot beads of melted synthetic material.

23. Tetanus
24. a. Compensate for water and sodium lost to traumatized areas and interstitial spaces
    b. Reestablish sodium balance
    c. Restore circulating volume
    d. Provide adequate perfusion
    e. Correct acidosis
    f. Improve renal function
25. Crystalloid solutions
26. High-protein, high-calorie diet
27. Vitamins A and C
28. Morphine sulfate
29. debridement
30. The water acts to loosen and remove sloughing tissue, exudate, and topical medications, cleanses the entire body, and aids in the maintenance of range of motion.
31. a. 3
    b. 4
    c. 1
    d. 5
    e. 2
32. F. Education related to fire safety and survival among young children should include practicing "stop, drop, and roll."
33. a. Stop the burning process
    b. Decrease the inflammatory response
    c. Rehydrate the skin
34. Sun protection factor of 15 allows them to remain in the sun 15 times 10, or 150 minutes.
35. Take the child to a health care facility with pediatric emergency treatment services for laboratory evaluation and surveillance.
36. a. Assessment
    b. Gastic decontamination
    c. Prevention of recurrence
37. Treat the child first, not the poison.
38. Ipecac
39. a. 2
    b. 1
    c. 4
    d. 3
    e. 5
    f. 6
    g. 7
40. Non-intact, lead-based paint or lead-contaminated soil
41. a. Poverty
    b. Being younger than 6 years of age
    c. Dwelling in urban areas
    d. Living in older rental homes, where lead decontamination may not be a priority

42. Neurologic system
43. Blood lead level test
44. Developmental delays, lowered intelligence quotient, reading skill deficits, visual-spatial problems, visual-motor problems, learning disabilities, and lower academic success; Physical growth and reproductive efficiency may also be adversely affected by chronic lead toxicity.
45. Prevention of initial or further exposure to lead
46. 681,000
47. Child neglect
48. Intracranial bleeding (subdural and subarachnoid hematomas) and bilateral retinal hemorrhages; fractures of the ribs and long bones. However, often there are no signs of external injury.
49. A rare but serious form of child abuse in which caregivers deliberately exaggerate or fabricate histories and symptoms or induce symptoms. It is a form of child maltreatment that may include physical, emotional, and psychologic abuse for the gratification of the caregiver.
50. F. Child maltreatment occurs across all socioeconomic groups.
51. a. Parental characteristics
    b. Characteristics of the child
    c. Environmental characteristics
52. a. Parental unavailability
    b. Lack of emotional closeness and flexibility
    c. Social isolation
    d. Emotional deprivation
    e. Communication difficulties
53. T

Applying Critical Thinking to the Nursing Practice

A.
1. Assessment should include developmental concerns, negative sleep associations, bedtime routines, media exposure, physical activities before bedtime, and cultural traditions including co-sleeping.
2. Interventions include limiting media time, ensuring all types of media are age appropriate and not too frightening or overstimulating, providing a consistent bedtime ritual, ignoring attention-seeking behavior and not allowing

Kim to stay up past her set bed time, providing a night light in Kim's room, using a favorite toy or blanket as a transitional object when going to bed, and promoting quiet time such as reading or bathing right before bed.

B.
1. Calamine lotion, soothing Burow solution compresses, or Aveeno baths for discomfort; topical corticosteroid gel for prevention or relief of inflammation; and oral corticosteroids for severe reactions. Benadryl may also be ordered for a sedative.
2. a. When the child has made contact with the plant, immediately flush the area with cold running water to neutralize the urushiol.
    b. Remove all clothing and thoroughly launder it in hot water and detergent.
    c. Prevent the child from scratching the lesions.

C.
1. In what year was the home built?
2. Permanent neurologic deficits, increased distractibility, short attention span, impulsivity, reading disabilities, and school failure
3. Identifying the sources of lead in the environment
4. The child's blood lead level and what it means; potential adverse health effects of an elevated blood lead level; sources of lead exposure and suggestions on how to reduce exposure; importance of wet cleaning to remove lead dust on floors, window sills, and other surfaces; importance of good nutrition in reducing the absorption and effects of lead; for persons with poor nutritional patterns, adequate intake of calcium and iron and importance of regular meals; need for follow-up testing to monitor the child's blood lead level; results of an environmental investigation, if applicable; hazards of improper removal of lead paint (dry sanding, scraping, or open-flame burning)

D.
1. a. Type of parenting received; negative relationship with own parents; social isolation;

low self-esteem; substance abuse; no support system; presence of concurrent stressors; inadequate knowledge of normal development; lack of knowledge of parenting skills; victims of child abuse themselves

b. Temperament; position in the family; age (between birth and 3 years old); additional physical or emotional needs; activity level; illegitimacy; reminding parents of someone they dislike; prematurity; product of difficult delivery; disabilities

c. Chronic stress from many sources, such as divorce, poverty, unemployment, poor housing, frequent relocation, alcoholism, overcrowding, and drug addiction

2. Any five of the following are acceptable:
- Conflicting stories about the accident or injury
- Cause of injury blamed on sibling or other party
- An injury inconsistent with the history
- History inconsistent with the child's developmental level
- A complaint other than the obvious injury
- Inappropriate response of caregiver
- Inappropriate response of child
- Repeated visits to emergency facilities with injuries

3. a. Risk for Trauma related to previous history of physical abuse, caregiver stress, and child's high level of energy

b. Fear/Anxiety related to maltreatment by mother, powerlessness, and potential loss of parent

c. Altered Parenting related to inadequate support, lack of education related to normal toddler behavior, and inadequate maternal coping skills

CHAPTER 14

Review of Essential Concepts

1. deciduous tooth, permanent teeth

2. F. Children grow an average of 5 cm (2 inches) per year and almost double their weight.

3. a. A decrease in head circumference in relation to standing height

b. A decrease in waist circumference in relation to height

c. An increase in leg length in relation to height

4. 10 years for girls, and 12 years for boys

5. d

6. d

7. inferiority

8. T

9. c

10. Conservation

11. numbers, substance

12. The ability to group and sort objects according to the attributes they share, place things in a sensible and logical order, and hold a concept in mind while making decisions based on that concept

13. T

14. d

15. b

16. peer

17. Peer group identification

18. a. To appreciate the various points of view found in the peer group

b. To become more sensitive to the social norms and pressures of the peer group

c. To form intimate friendships between same-sex peers

19. bullying

20. Bullying occurs most frequently at school where supervision is minimal, such as school hallways or on the playground.

21. division of labor

22. self-concept

23. T

24. Teachers

25. latchkey children

26. a. The psychosocial maturity of the parents

b. The childhood and childrearing experiences of the parents

c. The temperament of the children

d. The context of the children's misconduct

e. The response of the children to rewards and punishments

27. a. Stomach pains or headaches

b. Sleep problems

c. Bed-wetting

d. Changes in eating habits

e. Aggressive or stubborn behavior

f. Withdrawal or reluctance to participate in activities

g. Regression to earlier behaviors

h. Trouble concentrating or changes in academic performance

28. a. 1
b. 2
c. 2
d. 3
e. 1

29. Any of the following answers are appropriate:
- The easy availability of fast-food restaurants
- The influence of the mass media
- The temptation to eat "junk food"
- Sedentary lifestyles
- Easy availability of high-calorie foods

30. T

31. T

32. T

33. F. The most common cause of severe accidental injury and death in school-age children is motor vehicle accidents.

Applying Critical Thinking to the Nursing Practice

A.

1. a. Falls just below the 50th percentile
b. Falls at the 50th percentile

2. The nurse could explain to Ann that, at Cole's stage of development, he needs and wants real achievement. When he is recognized for his own unique talents and abilities and is positively rewarded, he will be able to achieve a sense of industry and accomplishment. Another important piece of information the nurse could offer Ann is that trying to make children into something or someone they are not often leads them to a sense of inferiority.

3. Lying, cheating, and stealing are frequent occurrences in the young school-age child. Children of this age often have difficulty

separating fact and fantasy. The nurse could inform Ann that it is important for her to teach her daughter the difference between fact and fantasy.

B.
1. Children at this age need to belong to a peer group, where they gain a sense of industry through individual and cooperative performance. It is necessary for school-age children to move away from the familiar relationships of the family group to increase the scope of interpersonal interactions and explore the environment. This is one way they gain the independence they will need to function as a healthy adult in society.
2. Children learn to appreciate the numerous and varied points of view that are represented in the peer group. As children interact with peers who see the world in ways that are somewhat different from their own, they become aware of the limits of their own point of view. Because age-mates are peers and are not forced to accept each other's ideas as they are expected to accept those of adults, other children have a significant influence on expanding the child's egocentric outlook. Consequently, children learn to argue, persuade, bargain, cooperate, and compromise in order to maintain friendships.
3. a. Instruct them on the proper use of seat belts while a passenger in a vehicle.
   b. Stress the importance of maintaining discipline while riding as a passenger in a vehicle (eg, keeping arms inside, not leaning against doors, not interfering with the driver).
   c. Remind the family that the child should never ride in the bed of a pickup truck.
   d. Teach the child safe pedestrian skills for crossing the road.
   e. Insist that the family as a group wear safety apparel (helmet when riding a bicycle, motorcycle, moped, or all-terrain vehicle).

4. a. Teach the child basic rules of water safety.
   b. Teach the family the importance of supervision when swimming.
   c. Teach the child and family to check sufficient water depth before diving.
   d. Teach the child to always swim with a companion.
   e. Insist that family members use an approved flotation device in water or on boats.
   f. Teach the child and family the importance of learning and being efficient in administering cardiopulmonary resuscitation.

CHAPTER 15

Review of Essential Concepts
1. 11 to 20, 13 to 19
2. a. Puberty is the maturational, hormonal, and growth processes that occur when the reproductive organs begin to function and secondary sex characteristics develop.
   b. Adolescence means "to grow into maturity" and is generally regarded as the psychologic, social, and maturational process initiated by the pubertal changes.
3. a. Increased physical growth
   b. Appearance and development of secondary sex characteristics
4. Primary sex characteristics
5. Secondary sex characteristics
6. Estrogen, androgens
7. Tanner stages
8. 10½ to 15 years; 12 years, 8 months for Caucasian girls and 12 years, 2 months for African-American girls
9. testicular, pubic hair
10. anterior pituitary gland, hypothalamus
11. Androgens
12. T
13. F
14. Identity formation
15. group
16. Because of the normal mood swings present in adolescence
17. Formal operations
18. a. Can imagine a sequence of events that might occur

   b. Is capable of scientific reasoning and formal logic
   c. Is capable of mentally manipulating more than two categories of variables at the same time
   d. Is able to detect logical consistencies or inconsistencies and can evaluate a system of values in a more analytic manner
   e. Is able to think about his or her own thinking and the thinking of others
19. Peer group
20. religiosity, spirituality
21. Authority is used to guide the adolescent while allowing developmentally appropriate levels of freedom and providing clear, consistent messages regarding expectations.
22. Sexual and substance-use behaviors
23. F
24. T
25. F
26. a. Injury
    b. Depression
    c. Eating disorders
    d. Substance use
    e. Sexually transmitted infections
    f. Pregnancy
    g. Obesity
27. T
28. a. Poor dietary habits
    b. Increasingly sedentary lifestyle
29. Meal patterns, dieting behaviors, consumption of high-fat and high-salt foods, recent weight changes
30. 60 minutes
31. Any five of the following are acceptable:
    • Body image
    • Sexuality conflicts
    • Academic pressures
    • Competitive pressures
    • Relationship with parents
    • Relationship with siblings
    • Relationship with peers
    • Finances
    • Decisions about present and future roles
    • Career planning
    • Ideologic conflicts
32. T
33. F
34. T

272

A.

1. a. Between the 50th and 75th percentiles
   b. At the 95th percentile
2. Non-lean body mass, primarily fat, increases in adolescence. Fatty tissue deposition is more pronounced in girls, particularly in the regions over the thighs, hips, buttocks, and breast tissue. Although the 95th percentile is the top of the normal range, nutritional counseling to prevent additional weight gain or eating disorders should be instituted. The nurse should also explain to Britney that adolescent acne is normal because of the hormonal changes she is currently experiencing. The nurse can observe Britney in her cleansing routine and point out ways to help decrease acne flare-ups.

B.

1. The peer group offers Billy a sense of group identity, which is essential to the later development of personal identity. Younger adolescents must resolve questions concerning relationships with a peer group before they are able to resolve questions about who they are in relation to the family and society.
2. Wearing clothes, makeup, and hairstyles according to group criteria; enjoying music and dancing exclusive to the age-group; using the same language; conforming to the peer group rather than to the adult world
3. They serve as a strong support to the adolescent, individually and collectively, providing a sense of belonging and a feeling of strength and power. They also form a transitional world between dependence and autonomy.

C.

1. Rapid physical growth, increased activity, poor nutrition, and a propensity for staying up late
2. Exercise for growing muscles, interactions with peers, competition, following rules of the game, socially acceptable means to enjoy stimulation and conflict

3. The need for independence and risk taking, feelings of indestructibility, and the need for peer approval

CHAPTER 16

Review of Essential Concepts

1. Enuresis
2. a. Medications
   b. Restriction or elimination of fluids after evening meal
   c. Avoidance of caffeinated and sugar-containing beverages after 4 pm
   d. Purposeful interruption of sleep to void
   e. Motivational therapy
   f. Devices to establish a conditioned reflex response (alarms)
3. F. Punishment is contraindicated because of its negative emotional impact and limited success in reducing the behavior.
4. Encopresis
5. Constipation
6. Psychogenic encopresis
7. boys, 6 and 8
8. 300 to 350
9. a. Absence of secondary sex characteristics and no uterine bleeding by 13 years of age, or absence of uterine bleeding with secondary sex characteristics by 16½ years of age
   b. Absence of menses after menstruation was previously established for at least 6 months in a woman with regular menstrual cycle or at least 12 months in a woman with irregular menstrual cycles
10. prostaglandins
11. Health teaching
12. Fluid retention, behavioral or emotional changes, premenstrual cravings, headache, fatigue, and backache
13. Diet including reduced consumption of refined sugar, salt, alcohol, and caffeinated beverages; three small- to moderate-sized meals with three small snacks rich in complex carbohydrates and fiber; exercise; and stress reduction
14. a. Increased condom use
    b. Increased contraception use
    c. Delayed initiation of sexual activity

15. a. Poor maternal weight gain
    b. Anemia
    c. Pregnancy-induced hypertension
16. Lack of awareness regarding one's susceptibility to sexually transmitted infections
17. Primary prevention consists of preventing infections while secondary prevention consists of prompt diagnosis and treatment of current infections.
18. a. 4, 10
    b. 1, 7
    c. 2, 8
    d. 5, 9
    e. 3, 6
19. T
20. Fever, chills, abdominal pain, nausea and vomiting, increased vaginal discharge, urinary tract symptoms, irregular bleeding
21. T
22. T
23. F. The primary goal of nursing care is to avoid inflicting further stress on the adolescent.
24. Body mass index
25. a. Elevated blood cholesterol
    b. High blood pressure
    c. Respiratory disorders
    d. Orthopedic conditions
    e. Cholelithiasis
    f. Some types of adult-onset cancer
    g. Nonalcoholic fatty liver disease
    h. Type 2 diabetes mellitus
26. Obesity
27. Mexican-American boys and non-Hispanic black girls
28. T
29. T
30. T
31. The refusal to maintain a minimally normal body weight and severe weight loss in the absence of obvious physical causes
32. a. Perfectionists
    b. Academically high achievers
    c. Conforming
    d. Conscientious
33. Any of the following are acceptable:
    a. Severe and profound weight loss
    b. Secondary or primary amenorrhea
    c. Sinus bradycardia
    d. Lowered body temperature

273

e. Hypotension
f. Cold intolerance
g. Dry skin and brittle nails
h. Appearance of lanugo hair and thinning hair
i. Abdominal pain, bloating, constipation
j. Fatigue
k. Lightheadedness
l. Evidence of muscle wasting (cachectic appearance)
m. Bone pain with exercise

34. a. Adolescent perception of high parental expectations for achievement and appearance
b. Difficulty managing conflict and poor communication styles
c. Enmeshment and occasionally estrangement between family members
d. Devaluation of the mother or the maternal role
e. Marital tension
f. Mood and anxiety disorders

35. Behavior of repeated episodes of binge eating followed by inappropriate compensatory behaviors, such as self-induced vomiting; misuse of laxatives, diuretics, or other medications; fasting; or excessive exercise

36. A distinct category that is similar to bulimia but purging is not involved

37. F. The female athlete triad is characterized by an eating disorder, amenorrhea, and osteoporosis

38. a. Treat any life-threatening malnutrition
b. Restore dietary stability and weight gain

39. With slow refeeding and the addition of phosphorus when total body phosphorus is depleted

40. Developmentally inappropriate degrees of inattention, impulsiveness, and hyperactivity

41. Psychiatric disorders, medical problems, and traumatic experiences

42. a. Medication
b. Family education and counseling
c. Psychotherapy
d. Environmental manipulation
e. Proper classroom placement

43. T
44. T

45. T
46. F. The primary goal of treating school phobia is school attendance.
47. Psychophysiologic disorder with a sudden onset that can usually be traced to a precipitating environmental event
48. Because children may be unable to express their feelings and tend to act out their problems and concerns rather than identifying them verbally
49. a. Predominantly sad facial expression with absence or diminished range of affective response
b. Solitary play, work, or tendency to be alone; disinterest in play
c. Withdrawal from previously enjoyed activities and relationships
d. Lowered grades in school; lack of interest in doing homework or achieving in school
e. Diminished motor activity; tiredness
f. Tearfulness or crying
g. Dependent and clinging or aggressive and disruptive behavior
50. T
51. Imitation of adult behavior; peer pressure; desire to imitate behaviors and lifestyles portrayed in movies and advertisements; desire to control weight
52. F. Smoking-prevention programs that focus on the negative, long-term effects of smoking on health have been ineffective.
53. a. Experimenters
b. Compulsive users
54. Changes to cognitive and autonomic functions such as judgment, memory, learning ability, and other intellectual capacities
55. sleep
56. Self-neglect of physical needs, overdose, contamination, and infection including HIV and hepatitis B and C infection
57. Because drug withdrawal can seriously complicate other illnesses
58. T
59. Suicidal ideation is a preoccupation with thoughts about

committing suicide and may be a precursor to suicide. Parasuicide refers to all behaviors ranging from gestures to serious attempts to kill oneself.
60. a. Early recognition
b. Management
c. Prevention

Applying Critical Thinking to the Nursing Practice

A.

1. Stress, changes in environment, weight changes, hyperandrogenism, eating disorders, and exercise-induced amenorrhea
2. a. Directly teach information about the disease to the patient.
b. Encourage abstinence or postponement of sexual intercourse; encourage condom use; advise to take hepatitis B vaccination and Gardasil (human papillomavirus quadrivalent) vaccine.
c. Decrease the medical and psychologic effects through support groups.

B.

1. Because it is obvious to others, is difficult to treat, and has long-term effects on psychologic and physical health status.
2. There is little evidence to support a relationship between obesity and "low metabolism." There may be small differences in regulation of dietary intake or metabolic rate between obese and non-obese children that could lead to an energy imbalance and inappropriate weight gain, but these small differences are difficult to accurately quantify.
3. a. Altered Nutrition: More Than Body Requirements, related to excess caloric intake, disordered eating patterns, hereditary factors, environmental conditions
b. Activity Intolerance related to sedentary lifestyle, physical bulk, pain on exertion
c. Ineffective Individual Coping related to little or no exercise, poor nutrition, personal vulnerability, body image disturbance

d. Self-Esteem Disturbance related to perception of physical appearance, internalization, or negative feedback

e. Altered Family Processes related to management of child who is obese, familial excessive caloric intake, lack of proper nutrition

C.

1. Dieting
2. The current emphasis on tall, thin individuals

D.

1. A history of family conflict; possibly a family history of suicide, depression, substance abuse, or emotional disturbance; parents who are unavailable and poor communicators. There is often also a history of unrealistically high parental expectations or parental indifference with low expectations.

2. Family support and counseling, having Becky sign a contract that she will not attempt another suicide, and individual counseling

CHAPTER 17

Review of Essential Concepts

1. a. Normalizing experiences
   b. Adapting the environment
   c. Promoting coping skills
2. communication, negotiation
3. negative psychologic effects
4. a. Disrespectful attitudes
   b. Breaking bad news in an insensitive manner
   c. Withholding information
   d. Changing a treatment course without preparing the child and family
5. Developing a care plan in conjunction with the family while considering their preferences and priorities
6. a. The time of diagnosis
   b. During the initial discharge home
7. a. Accept the child's condition.
   b. Manage the child's condition on a day-to-day basis.
   c. Meet the child's normal developmental needs.
   d. Meet the developmental needs of other family members.
   e. Cope with ongoing stress and periodic crises.

f. Assist family members in managing their feelings.
   g. Educate others about the child's condition.
   h. Establish a support system.

8. Any two of the following are acceptable:
   • Value each child individually and avoid comparisons.
   • Remind each child of his or her positive qualities and contribution to other family members.
   • Help siblings see differences and similarities between themselves and the child with special needs.
   • Create a climate in which children can achieve success without feeling guilty.
   • Teach siblings ways to interact with the child.
   • Seek to be fair in terms of discipline, attention, and resources.
   • Let siblings settle their own differences; intervene only to prevent siblings from hurting one another.
   • Legitimize reasonable anger.
   • Respect a sibling's reluctance to be with or to include the child with special needs in activities.

9. A process of recognizing, promoting, and enhancing competence

10. Any three of the following are acceptable:
    • Physician shopping
    • Attributing the symptoms of the actual illness to a minor condition
    • Refusing to believe the diagnostic tests
    • Delaying consent for treatment
    • Acting happy and optimistic despite the revealed diagnosis
    • Refusing to tell or talk to anyone about the condition
    • Insisting that no one is telling the truth, regardless of others' attempts to do so
    • Denying the reason for admission
    • Asking no questions about the diagnosis, treatment, or prognosis

11. a. Guilt
    b. Self-accusation

c. Bitterness
   d. Anger
12. a. 4
    b. 3
    c. 2
    d. 1
13. a. Available support system
    b. Perception of the event
    c. Coping mechanisms
    d. Reactions to the child
    e. Available resources
    f. Concurrent stresses within the family
14. F. The level of adjustment is significantly influenced by the functional burden on the family.
15. T
16. T
17. a. Feels different and withdraws
    b. Is irritable, is moody, and acts out
18. It can produce increased participation in health-seeking behaviors and an improved sense of well-being.
19. F. Children with more severe disorders often cope better than those with milder conditions.
20. Because factors affecting the family's response may change at any point during the illness
21. b
22. By presenting the child's strengths, appealing behaviors, and potential for development
23. Encourage children to express their concerns rather than allowing others to express them for them
24. Educating the family about the disorder
25. Encourage the child's self-care abilities in both activities of daily living and medical regimen
26. realistic future goals
27. body changes
28. a. Developmental factors
    b. Medical advances and technology
    c. Changing social patterns
29. To live life to the fullest without pain, with choices and dignity, in the familiar environment of their home, and with the support of their family
30. Euthanasia involves an action carried out by a person other than the patient to end the life of the patient suffering from a terminal condition. The intent

of this action is based on the belief that the act is "putting the person out of his or her misery"; this action has also been called mercy killing. Assisted suicide, on the other hand, occurs when someone provides the patient with the means to end his or her life and the patient uses that means to do so.

31. a. Fear of pain and suffering
    b. Fear of dying alone (child) or of not being present when the child dies (parent)
    c. Fear of actual death
32. Cheyne-Stokes; that this breathing is not distressing to the child and that it is a normal part of the dying process
33. T
34. F. Grief is a process, not an event. It is not orderly or predictable.
35. T
36. d
37. Any of the four following responses can apply:
    a. Maintaining good general health
    b. Developing well-rounded interests
    c. Using distancing techniques, such as taking time off when needed
    d. Developing and using professional and personal support systems
    e. Cultivating the capacity for empathy
    f. Focusing on the positive aspects of the caregiver role
    g. Basing nursing interventions on sound theory and empiric observations
    h. Attending shared-remembrance rituals or funeral services

Applying Critical Thinking to the Nursing Practice

A.
1. Children need honest and accurate information about their illness, treatments, and prognosis using clear, simple language and appropriate information about the disease, illness, and possible death.
2. When the prognosis for a patient is poor, and death is the expected outcome.

B.
1. Home care represents the return to a system and set of priorities in which family values are as important in the care of a child with a chronic health problem as they are in the care of other children.
2. a. Normalize the life of the child, including those with technologically complex care, in a family and community context and setting.
   b. Minimize the disruptive impact of the child's condition on the family.
   c. Foster the child's maximum growth and development.

C.
1. a. Status of the marital relationship
   b. Alternate support systems
   c. Ability to communicate
2. This assists in the ability to evaluate the individual's coping patterns with various aspects of the crisis and identifies possible areas for intervention.
3. Could be any of the following:
   a. "Competence and optimism" involves an accentuation on positive aspects of the situation; child concentrates more on what he/she can do rather than what is missing or what he/she cannot do
   b. "Feels different and withdraws" involves the child seeing him/herself as different from other children in a way that is negative; focuses on things he/she cannot do and sometimes overrestricts activities
   c. "Complies with treatment" involves the child taking necessary medications and treatments; adheres to activity restrictions
   d. "Seeks support" involves the child talking with adults, children, physicians, or nurses; develops a plan to handle problems as they occur
4. a. Provide support at the time of diagnosis.
   b. Accept the family's emotional reactions.
   c. Support the family's coping methods.
   d. Educate about the disorder and general health care.

   e. Establish an environment of normalization for the child.
   f. Establish realistic future goals.

D.
1. Answers may vary.
   a. May view death as a departure like sleep
   b. May recognize the fact of physical death but fail to separate it from living
   c. May view death as temporary, as though life and death can change places
   d. May have no understanding of the universality and inevitability of death
2. As punishment for his or her behavior
3. 9 to 10 years
4. a. Help parents deal with their feelings.
   b. Avoid alliances with either parent or child.
   c. Structure hospital admission to allow for maximum self-control and independence.
   d. Answer the adolescent's questions honestly and treat them with respect.
   e. Help parents understand child's reactions to death and dying.

E.
1. a. Providing detailed information about what will happen if supportive equipment is withdrawn
   b. Ensuring that appropriate pain medications are administered to prevent pain during the dying process
   c. Allowing the parents time before the start of the withdrawal to be with and speak to their child
2. a. Providing privacy
   b. Asking whether they would like to play music
   c. Softening lights and monitor noises
   d. Arranging for any religious or cultural rituals that the family may want performed
3. After the child's death, the family should be allowed to remain with the body and hold or rock the child if they desire. After the nurse has removed all tubes and equipment from the body,

parents should be given the option of assisting with the preparation of the body, such as bathing and dressing. It is important for the nurse to determine whether the family has any specific needs, since many cultures have adapted specific methods for coping and mourning death, and impeding these practices may interfere with the grieving process.

4. If there is a full-time transplant coordinator, the nurse's role is to contact that coordinator to meet with the family. If such services are not available, the staff needs to determine which members should discuss this topic with the family. Often nurses are in an optimal position to suggest tissue donation after consultation with the attending physician. When possible, the topic should be raised before death occurs. The request should be made in a private and quiet area of the hospital and should be simple and direct, with questions such as "Are you a donor family?" or "Have you ever considered organ donation?"

5. The family may have an open casket, and there is no delay in the funeral. There is no cost to the donor family, but organ donation does not eliminate funeral or cremation responsibilities.

CHAPTER 18

Review of Essential Concepts

1. c
2. d
3. Any three of the following:
    a. Dysmorphic syndromes (eg, Down syndrome, fragile X syndrome)
    b. Irritability or nonresponsiveness to environment
    c. Major organ system dysfunction (eg, feeding or breathing difficulties)
    d. Gross motor delay
    e. Fine motor delay
    f. Language difficulties or delay
    g. Behavior difficulties
4. Developmental disability
5. b
6. d
7. c

8. a. A task analysis of the individual steps needed to master a skill must be done before teaching.
    b. Observing the child to determine what skills are possessed and the child's developmental readiness to learn the task.
9. b
10. b
11. a
12. T
13. b
14. a. Hearing impaired is a general term indicating disability that may range in severity from mild to profound and includes the subsets of deaf and hard-of-hearing.
    b. Deaf refers to a person whose hearing disability precludes successful processing of linguistic information through audition, with or without a hearing aid.
    c. Hard-of-hearing refers to a person who, generally with the use of a hearing aid, has residual hearing sufficient to enable successful processing of linguistic information through audition.
15. Conductive or middle-ear hearing loss results from interference of transmission of sound to the middle ear. It is the most common of all types of hearing loss and most frequently is a result of recurrent serous otitis media. Sensorineural hearing loss, also called perceptive or nerve deafness, involves damage to the inner ear structures or the auditory nerve. Sensorineural hearing loss results in distortion of sound, severely affecting discrimination and comprehension.
16. hearing aid
17. a
18. a. An inability to express ideas in any form, either written or verbal
    b. The inability to interpret sound correctly
    c. Difficulty in processing details or discriminating among sounds
19. a
20. c
21. a. 2, 4, 8
    b. 1, 7, 10

c. 5, 9
    d. 3, 6
22. d
23. b
24. Look for blinking. Also check to see whether the infant's activity level accelerates or slows or respiratory patterns change when an object comes near; also check to see whether the infant makes throaty sounds when the parents speak to him or her.
25. Through finger spelling
26. They interfere with the normal sequence of physical, intellectual, and psychosocial growth.
27. c
28. Inability to engage in social interactions, communication difficulties, and behavior problems
29. F

Applying Critical Thinking to the Nursing Practice

A.

1. Dysmorphic features of Down syndrome or fragile X syndrome, irritability or unresponsiveness to contact, abnormal eye contact during feeding, gross motor delay, decreased alertness to voice or movement, language difficulties or delay, feeding difficulties

2. For each body system, any two of the following are acceptable.
    a. Head and eyes: separated sagittal suture, brachycephaly, rounded and small skull, flat occiput, enlarged anterior fontanel, oblique palpebral fissures, inner epicanthal folds, speckling of iris
    b. Nose and ears: small nose, depressed nasal bridge, small ears and narrow canals, short pinna, overlapping upper helices, conductive hearing loss
    c. Mouth and neck: high, arched, narrow palate; protruding tongue; hypoplastic mandible; delayed teeth eruption and microdontia; abnormalities in tooth alignment; periodontal disease; neck skin excess and laxity; short and broad neck
    d. Chest and heart: shortened rib cage, twelfth rib anomalies, pectus excavatum, congenital heart defects

e. Abdomen and genitalia: protruding, lax, and flabby abdominal muscles; diastasis recti abdominis; umbilical hernia; small penis; cryptorchidism; bulbous vulva

f. Hands and feet: broad, short hands and stubby fingers; incurved little finger; transverse palmar crease; wide space between big and second toes; plantar crease between big and second toes; broad, short feet and stubby toes

g. Musculoskeletal system and skin: short stature; hyperflexibility and muscle weakness; hypotonia; atlantoaxial instability; dry, cracked skin and frequent fissuring; cutis marmorata (mottling)

h. Other: reduced birth weight, learning difficulty, hypothyroidism, impaired immune function, increased risk of leukemia

3. a. Ensure that the parents are informed as soon as possible after the birth of the child.

b. Encourage parents to be together at this time to emotionally support each other.

c. Provide parents with written material concerning the syndrome when they are ready to receive it.

d. Offer referrals to parent groups or professional counseling.

B.

1. Perinatal infections (herpes, chlamydia, gonococci, rubella, syphilis, toxoplasmosis); retinopathy of prematurity; trauma; postnatal infections (meningitis); and disorders such as sickle cell disease, juvenile rheumatoid arthritis, Tay-Sachs disease, albinism, and retinoblastoma. In many instances, such as with refractive errors, the cause of the defect is unknown.

2. a. One intervention is assessing parents' concerns regarding visual responsiveness in their child such as lack of eye contact from the infant. Another intervention is to test for strabismus. Lack of binocularity after 4 months of age is considered abnormal and must be treated to prevent amblyopia. The nurse should also observe the neonate's response to visual stimuli, such as following a light or object, and cessation of body movement.

b. Because the most common visual impairment during childhood is refractive errors, testing for visual acuity is essential. The school nurse usually assumes major responsibility for vision testing in schoolchildren. In addition to refractive errors, the nurse should be aware of signs and symptoms that indicate other ocular problems. Additional interventions include educating parents on how to prevent sports-related injuries and infections, identifying behaviors that suggest visual problems, and identifying children who are at risk because of genetic factors.

3. a. Tapping method (use of a cane to survey the environment for direction and to avoid obstacles)

b. Guides such as a sighted human guide or a dog guide (such as a seeing eye dog)

4. a. Help parents identify clues other than eye contact from the infant that signify communication.

b. Encourage parents to show affection using nonvisual methods, such as talking, reading, cuddling, or massaging the infant.

C.

Show them a picture of a child with an eye prosthesis. Prepare them for the appearance of the wound. Within 3 weeks the child will be fitted for a prosthesis, and the facial appearance will return to normal. Care of the socket is minimal and easily accomplished.

D.

1. The majority (50% to 70%) have some degree of cognitive impairment.

2. Early recognition of behaviors associated with autism spectrum disorders, including speech and language delays, no babbling by 12 months, single words by 16 months, two-word phrases by 24 months, and a sudden deterioration in extant expressive speech

3. Those with communicative speech development by age 6 and an intelligence quotient above 50 at the time of diagnosis

CHAPTER 19

Review of Essential Concepts

1. c
2. c
3. separation anxiety
4. Temper tantrum, anger expressions, bed-wetting
5. F
6. d
7. a. 1
   b. 2
   c. 1
   d. 3
   e. 4
8. b
9. a. "Difficult" temperament
   b. Lack of fit between child and parent
   c. Age (especially between 6 months and 5 years)
   d. Male gender
   e. Below-average intelligence
   f. Multiple and continuing stresses (eg, frequent hospitalizations)
10. T
11. Feeling an overall sense of helplessness, questioning the skills of staff, accepting the reality of hospitalization, needing to have information explained in simple language, dealing with fear, coping with uncertainty, seeking reassurance from caregivers
12. b
13. unknown, known
14. d
15. separation
16. This care recognizes the integral role of the family in a child's life and acknowledges the family as an essential part of the child's care and illness experience. The family is considered to be partners in the child's care.
17. a. Promote freedom of movement.
    b. Maintain the child's routine.
    c. Encourage independence.
    d. Promote understanding.

18. b
19. c
20. The nurse repeatedly stressing the reason for a procedure and evaluating the child's understanding
21. It is important not to use this terminology with children because it often leads to greater fears in hospitalized children.
22. a. By providing a somewhat different and less negative account of the disease
    b. By offering an explanation that is characteristic of the next stage of cognitive development
23. T
24. a. The nurse can encourage children to resume schoolwork as quickly as their condition permits.
    b. The nurse can help them schedule and protect a selected time for studies.
    c. The nurse can help the family coordinate hospital educational services with their children's schools.
25. d
26. Any three of the following:
    • Provides diversion and promotes relaxation
    • Helps the child feel more secure in a strange environment
    • Helps reduce the stress of separation and feeling of homesickness
    • Provides a means for release of tension and expression of feelings
    • Encourages interaction and development of positive attitudes toward others
    • Provides an expression outlet for creative ideas and interests
    • Provides a means for accomplishing therapeutic goals
    • Places child in active role and provides opportunity to make choices and be in control
27. a
28. a. 4
    b. 1
    c. 2
    d. 3

29. Any two of the following are correct:
    a. Fostering parent-child relationships
    b. Providing educational opportunities
    c. Promoting self-mastery
    d. Providing socialization
30. c
31. a. Minimization of the stressors of hospitalization
    b. Reduced chance of infection
    c. Cost savings
32. Giving simple explanations, such as "You need to be in this room to help you get better."
33. T

Applying Critical Thinking to the Nursing Practice

A.
1. protest
2. despair
3. Any one of the following is acceptable:
    • Allow Paul to cry or encourage the child to express his feelings.
    • When Paul withdraws, encourage the parents to continue to move toward him and attempt to get him to play or communicate with them.
    • Provide support through physical presence in the room even when Paul rejects strangers.
    • Acknowledge to Paul that it is all right to miss his parents and it is all right to cry.
    • Encourage the parents to stay with Paul as much as possible.
    • Parents should let Paul know when they are leaving and when they will be returning.
    • Parents should bring favorite articles from home to comfort Paul.

B.
1. Regression
2. Any three of the following are acceptable:
    • Encourage her to perform all the self-care activities she can.
    • Provide positive feedback for the activities Kristi performs on her own.
    • Give Kristi two choices whenever possible.

• Encourage Kristi to freely express her needs, ideas, and feelings.
• Try to make Kristi's routine as consistent and familiar as possible.
• Minimize the restraint of physical activity.

C.
1. Any three of the following are acceptable:
    • Respect parental rights, values, beliefs, and individuality.
    • Convey an attitude of caring concern for both child and family.
    • Support and emphasize the family's strengths and abilities.
    • Provide feedback and praise.
    • Refer to other professionals for additional support.
    • Create an atmosphere of shared communication, respect, trust, and openness.
    • Serve as a family advocate.
    • Provide continuity of care.
2. Any three of the following are acceptable:
    • Recognize that family members know the child best and are "cued in" to the child's needs.
    • Allow the family to have unlimited presence.
    • Encourage family to bring siblings and other family members to visit.
    • Encourage family to provide the child with significant but manageable items from home.
    • Arrange for family members to have a meal together.
    • Attempt to make the hospital environment as much like home as possible.
3. Games such as puzzles; illustrated books; quiet, individual activities; Lego blocks and other building materials

CHAPTER 20

Review of Essential Concepts

1. It is the legal and ethical requirement that the patient or the patient's legal surrogate receive sufficient information on which to make an informed health care decision. The patient must also

demonstrate a clear, full, and complete understanding of the medical treatment to be performed and all risks of treatment and nontreatment before giving informed consent.

2. a. The person must be capable of giving consent, must be over the age of majority (usually age 18), and must be considered competent.
   b. The person must receive the information needed to make an intelligent decision.
   c. The person must act voluntarily when exercising freedom of choice, without force, fraud, deceit, duress, or other forms of constraint or coercion.

3. F
4. c
5. a. Imagery
   b. Distraction
   c. Relaxation
6. F
7. a
8. a
9. therapeutic
10. a. 3
    b. 2
    c. 1
    d. 4
11. c
12. If children have no preoperative pain and are well prepared psychologically for surgery
13. d
14. a
15. b
16. Any of the following three are correct:
    a. Impaired mobility
    b. Protein malnutrition
    c. Edema
    d. Incontinence
    e. Sensory loss
    f. Anemia
    g. Infection
    h. Not turning the patient
    i. Intubation
17. b
18. amount, tissue damage
19. c
20. F
21. c
22. c
23. a. 3
    b. 1
    c. 2

24. a. T
    b. F
    c. F
    d. T
    e. F
25. Entrapment when it is activated to descend
26. b
27. c
28. a. Combine the major features of universal precautions and body substance isolation; designed for use with all patients, especially those who are undiagnosed; involve the use of barrier protection such as gloves, masks, and gowns
    b. Used for patients known or suspected to be infected with epidemiologically important pathogens for which additional precautions beyond standard precautions are needed to interrupt transmission in hospitals; include airborne, droplet, and contact precautions
29. Handwashing
30. Any means, physical or mechanical, that restricts a person's movement, physical activity, or normal access to his or her body
31. T
32. Maintain the child's spine in a flexed position by holding the child with one arm behind the neck and the other behind the thighs.
33. c
34. urinary tract infection
35. F
36. Because they have immature enzyme systems in the liver (where most drugs are metabolized and detoxified), lower plasma concentrations of protein for binding with drugs, and immaturely functioning kidneys (where most drugs are excreted).
37. body surface area
38. a. Vastus lateralis muscle
    b. Ventrogluteal muscle
39. T
40. Blowing a small puff of air in the face
41. F
42. Any two of the following is correct:
    a. Inability to differentiate one type of loss from another because of admixture

    b. Loss of urine or liquid stool from leakage or evaporation (especially if the infant is under a radiant warmer)
    c. Additional fluid in the diaper (superabsorbent disposable type) from absorption of atmospheric moisture
43. Intraosseous infusion
44. retina, lungs
45. It is a physiologic hazard of oxygen therapy that may occur in persons with chronic pulmonary disease, such as cystic fibrosis. In these patients, the respiratory center has adapted to the continuously higher arterial carbon dioxide tension ($Paco_2$) levels, and therefore hypoxia becomes the more powerful stimulus for respiration.
46. a. Oximetry does not require heating the skin, thus reducing the risk of burns.
    b. Oximetry eliminates a delay period for transducer equilibration.
    c. Oximetry maintains an accurate measurement regardless of the patient's age or skin characteristics or the presence of lung disease.
47. T
48. c
49. humidified
50. respiratory, cardiac
51. It is used to check for proper placement.
52. postpyloric
53. Any three of the following are acceptable:
    • Carbohydrates
    • Lipids
    • Amino acids
    • Vitamins
    • Minerals
    • Water
    • Trace elements and other additives in a single container
    • Protein
    • Glucose
54. a. Osmotic effect of the enema may produce diarrhea, which can lead to metabolic acidosis.
    b. Extreme hyperphosphatemia, hypernatremia, and hypocalcemia can occur, which may lead to neuromuscular irritability and coma.
55. d

Applying Critical Thinking to the Nursing Practice

A.

1. Measure the rectal temperature 30 minutes after the antipyretic is given to assess whether the temperature is lowered.

2. Having the child wear minimal clothing; exposing the skin to the air; reducing room temperature; increasing air circulation; and applying cool, moist compresses to the skin (eg, the forehead) are effective if employed approximately 1 hour after an antipyretic is given so that the set point is lowered.

3. Parents should know how to take the child's temperature and read the thermometer accurately. They also need instruction in administering the drug. Emphasize accuracy in both the amount of drug given and the time intervals at which the drug is administered.

B.

1. Ensure the order is renewed daily; monitor the patient at least every 2 hours for signs of irritation, redness, or swelling around the restraints; remove restraints every 2 hours to exercise arms and joints; frequently monitor and assess his nutrition and hydration, circulation and range-of-motion of extremities, vital signs, hygiene and elimination, physical and psychologic status and comfort, and readiness for discontinuation of restraint.

2. Restraints with ties must be secured to the bed or crib frame, not the side rails. Leave one finger breadth between skin and the device; tie knots that allow for quick release; ensure the restraint does not tighten as the child moves; decrease wrinkles or bulges in the restraint; place jacket restraints over an article of clothing; place limb restraints below waist level, below knee level, or distal to the IV; and tuck in dangling straps.

C.

1. a. Talk often to Evan so that he knows someone is always nearby.
   b. Place a familiar toy inside the tent.
   c. Remove Evan from the tent for feeding and bathing if medically stable.

2. For infants, special devices are available for percussing small areas. A "popping," hollow sound should be the result, not a slapping sound. The procedure should be done over the rib cage only and should be painless.

3. The nurse would auscultate the chest before treatment and then after treatment to hear whether the chest sounds are clearer.

D.

1. Hemorrhage, edema, aspiration, accidental decannulation, tube obstruction, and the entrance of free air into the pleural cavity

2. Maintaining a patent airway, facilitating the removal of pulmonary secretions, providing humidified air or oxygen, cleansing the stoma, monitoring the child's ability to swallow, and teaching while simultaneously preventing complications

3. Noisy breathing, bubbling, or coughing

4. To prevent hypoxia

CHAPTER 21

Review of Essential Concepts

1. Respiratory tract infections
2. a. Age of the child
   b. Season
   c. Living conditions
   d. Preexisting medical problems
3. The diameter of the airways is smaller in children and is subject to considerable narrowing from edematous mucous membranes and increased production of secretions. The distance between structures within the respiratory tract is also shorter in the young child, and organisms may move rapidly down the respiratory tract, causing more extensive involvement. The relatively short and open Eustachian tube in infants and young children allows pathogens easy access to the middle ear.
4. a. T
   b. T
   c. T
   d. F. Vomiting is common in small children with illness.
   e. F. Abdominal pain is a common complaint.

5. Running a shower of hot water into the empty bathtub or open shower stall with the bathroom door closed produces a quick source of steam. Keeping a child in this environment for 10 to 15 minutes humidifies inspired air and can help relieve symptoms.

6. Apply 2 to 3 drops of saline (which can be prepared at home by dissolving 1 teaspoon of salt in 1 cup of warm water) into the child's nares and suction with a bulb syringe.

7. a. 1, 2, 5, 6, 7
   b. 3, 4, 8

8. No. Over-the-counter cold preparations such as pseudoephedrine and some antihistamines may cause serious side effects and have been associated with death in infants.

9. To differentiate between a viral and bacterial throat infection

10. Oral penicillin V or amoxicillin for 10 days

11. 24 hours, a full 24-hour period

12. Tonsils

13. A child who has difficulty swallowing and breathing and therefore breathes through his or her mouth

14. a. Recurrent throat infections (seven or more episodes in the preceding year; five or more episodes in each of the preceding 2 years; or three or more episodes in each of the preceding 3 years)
    b. Sleep-disordered breathing

15. Postoperative hemorrhage

16. Because it is associated with Reye syndrome.

17. a. An inflammation of the middle ear without reference to etiology or pathogenesis
    b. A rapid onset of signs and symptoms of acute infection, specifically fever and otalgia (ear pain)
    c. Fluid in the middle ear space without symptoms of acute infection

18. Purulent discolored effusion and a bulging or full, opacified, or reddened immobile membrane

19. 72 hours

20. Oral amoxicillin in high doses (80 to 90 mg/kg/day divided twice daily)
21. Routine immunization with pneumococcal conjugate vaccine (Prevnar 7)
22. Herpes-like Epstein-Barr virus
23. a. Headache
    b. Epistaxis
    c. Malaise
    d. Fatigue
    e. Chills
    f. Low-grade fever
    g. Loss of appetite
    h. Puffy eyes
24. Monospot is a rapid, sensitive, inexpensive, and easy-to-perform test, and it has the advantage that it can detect significant agglutinins at lower levels, thus allowing earlier diagnosis. Blood is usually obtained for the test by finger puncture and is placed on special paper. If the blood agglutinates, forming fragments or clumps, the test is positive for the infection.
25. Breathing difficulties, severe abdominal pain, sore throat so severe the child cannot eat or drink, and respiratory stridor
26. Hoarseness, a resonant cough described as "barking" or "brassy," varying degrees of inspiratory stridor, and varying degrees of respiratory distress resulting from swelling or obstruction in the region of the larynx and subglottic airway
27. A serious obstructive inflammatory process of the supraglottic
28. a. Absence of spontaneous cough
    b. Drooling
    c. Agitation
29. a. The voice is thick and muffled, with a froglike croaking sound on inspiration, but the child is not hoarse.
    b. Suprasternal and substernal retractions may be evident. The child seldom struggles to breathe, and slow, quiet breathing provides better air exchange.
    c. The sallow color of mild hypoxia may progress to frank cyanosis if treatment is delayed.
    d. The throat is red and inflamed, and a distinctive large, cherry-red, edematous epiglottis is visible on careful throat inspection.
30. It could precipitate a spasm of the epiglottis and complete obstruction of the airway.
31. Acute laryngotracheobronchitis
32. T
33. T
34. Respiratory syncytial virus affects the epithelial cells of the respiratory tract. The ciliated cells swell, protrude into the lumen, and lose their cilia. The walls of the bronchi and bronchioles are infiltrated with inflammatory cells, and varying degrees of intraluminal obstruction lead to hyperinflation, obstructive emphysema resulting from partial obstruction, and patchy areas of atelectasis.
35. T
36. Droplet and standard precautions
37. Etiologic agent
38. Any three of the following are acceptable:
    • *M. pneumoniae*
    • *Chlamydia pneumoniae*
    • *M. tuberculosis*
    • respiratory viruses
39. bulb suction syringe, mechanical suction, or nasal aspirator
40. Pertussis
41. Mycobacterium tuberculosis
42. airway
43. a. Adequate nutrition
    b. Pharmacotherapy
    c. General supportive measures
    d. Prevention of unnecessary exposure to other infections
    e. Prevention of reinfection
    f. Sometimes surgical procedures
44. Airborne precautions, negative-pressure room
45. avoid contact
46. compliance
47. T
48. a. Dyspnea
    b. Cough
    c. Stridor
    d. Hoarseness
49. Bronchoscopy
50. a. Abdominal thrusts for children older than 1 year of age
    b. Back blows and chest thrusts for children younger than 1 year of age
51. c
52. F. Acute respiratory distress syndrome may occur in both children and adults.
53. Increased respiratory illnesses, increased respiratory symptoms, and reduced performance on pulmonary function tests
54. a. Worsening air pollution
    b. More premature infants with chronic lung disease
    c. Poor access to medical care
    d. Underdiagnosis
    e. Undertreatment
55. a. T
    b. T
56. b and d
57. a. Long-term control medications are used to achieve and maintain control of inflammation.
    b. Quick-relief medications are used to treat symptoms and exacerbations.
58. Corticosteroids
59. Beta-adrenergic agonists
60. Both help to produce physical and mental relaxation, improve posture, strengthen respiratory musculature, and develop more efficient patterns of breathing.
61. Exercise-induced bronchospasm is an acute, reversible, usually self-terminating airway obstruction that develops during or after vigorous activity, reaches its peak 5 to 10 minutes after stopping the activity, and usually stops in another 20 to 30 minutes.
62. It is not recommended for allergens that can be eliminated, such as foods, drugs, and animal dander.
63. An asthma attack in which the child continues to display respiratory distress despite vigorous therapeutic measures
64. Inhaled aerosolized short-acting beta2-agonists and systemic corticosteroids. If the child is not responding, intravenous magnesium sulfate may also be given.
65. a. Provide effective communication.
    b. Assess the child and family's satisfaction with asthma control and quality of care.
    c. Assess the child and family's perception of severity of disease and social support.

66. a. Rhinorrhea
    b. Cough
    c. Low-grade fever
    d. Irritability
    e. Itching (especially in front of the neck and chest)
    f. Apathy
    g. Anxiety
    h. Sleep disturbance
    i. Abdominal discomfort
    j. Loss of appetite
67. a. Increased viscosity of mucous gland secretions
    b. A striking elevation of sweat electrolytes
    c. An increase in several organic and enzymatic constituents of saliva
    d. Abnormalities in autonomic nervous system function
68. mechanical obstruction
69. The first manifestation of cystic fibrosis in which the small intestine is blocked with thick, puttylike, tenacious, mucilaginous meconium
70. Because essential pancreatic enzymes are unable to reach the duodenum, digestion and absorption of nutrients are markedly impaired.
71. Bulky stools that are frothy and foul-smelling
72. Rectal prolapse
73. sodium, chloride
74. Improving ventilation, removing mucopurulent secretions, administering antimicrobial agents
75. a. Beginning of all meals and snacks
    b. Severity of insufficiency, how the child's body responds to enzyme therapy, and the practitioner's philosophy
    c. Normal growth and reduction in stools to one or at the most two per day
76. Well-balanced, high-protein, high-calorie diet supplemented with multivitamins and vitamins A, D, E, and K
77. Lung, heart, pancreas, and liver transplantation
78. a. Nightly snoring
    b. Labored breathing during sleep
    c. Interrupted or disturbed sleep patterns
    d. Sleep enuresis
    e. Daytime neurobehavioral problems

79. adenotonsillectomy
80. a. Increased work of breathing but with gas exchange function near normal
    b. Inability to maintain normal blood gas tensions and development of hypoxemia and acidosis as result of carbon dioxide retention
81. Respiratory arrest is the cessation of respiration; apnea is the cessation of breathing for more than 20 seconds or a shorter amount of time when associated with hypoxemia or bradycardia.
82. Restlessness, tachypnea, tachycardia, diaphoresis
83. a. F. Blind finger sweeps are avoided in all infants and children.
    b. F. The victim should not be moved in any way if trauma is suspected and should not be placed in the recovery position.

Applying Critical Thinking to the Nursing Practice

A.
1. Any two of the following are acceptable:
   • Ineffective Breathing Pattern related to inflammatory process
   • Fear/Anxiety related to difficulty breathing, unfamiliar procedures, and possibly environment (hospital)
   • Ineffective Airway Clearance related to mechanical obstruction, inflammation, increased secretions, pain
   • Risk for Infection related to presence of infective organisms
   • Activity Intolerance related to inflammatory process, imbalance between oxygen supply and demand
   • Pain related to inflammatory process, surgical incision
   • Altered Family Process related to illness or hospitalization of a child
   • Altered Nutrition: Less Than Body Requirements related to illness or hospitalization of the child
2. a. Warm or cool mist in the form of a mist tent or warm shower
   b. Instillation of saline nose drops to clear nasal passages

B.
1. Waiting up to 72 hours for spontaneous resolution is safe and appropriate management of acute otitis media in healthy infants over 6 months and in children
2. Irritability, crying, fussiness, pulling on her ears or rolling her head from side to side, complaining of pain, low-grade fever to as much as 40° C (104° F), anorexia, and signs of respiratory or pharyngeal infection

C.
1. On the basis of clinical manifestations, an absolute increase in atypical lymphocytes, and a positive Monospot test
2. The mechanism of spread is not understood completely, but it is believed to be transmitted in saliva by direct intimate contact.
3. The nurse could explain to Jenna that a drop of blood obtained by finger puncture will be placed on special paper. If the blood agglutinates, forming fragments or clumps, the test is positive for the infection.
4. a. To relieve the symptoms
   b. To establish appropriate activities according to stage of disease and her interests

D.
1. Acute laryngotracheobronchitis
2. When Billy became unable to inhale a sufficient volume of air and exhale carbon dioxide because of his narrowing airway
3. Respiratory acidosis and eventually respiratory failure
4. Continuous, vigilant observation and accurate assessment of respiratory status; keeping child calm (near parents) and quiet
5. Provides relief by decreasing edema of the respiratory tract

E.
1. Because of concerns about the high cost, aerosol route of administration, potential toxic effects among exposed health care personnel, and conflicting results of efficacy trials
2. Encourage his mother to continue nursing him often. If needed, it is also important to help the breastfeeding mother in pumping milk and storing it appropriately.

283

F.

1. Hacking, nonproductive cough; shortness of breath
2. Shortness of breath; productive cough; audible wheezing; deep, dark red color to the lips; cyanosis; restlessness and apprehension; sweating; use of accessory muscles; rapid respirations; upright position with hunched shoulders; speaking with short, panting, broken phrases; wheezes throughout lung fields; prolonged expiration; and crackles
3. a. Relief of bronchospasm
   b. Irritability, tremor, nervousness, and insomnia
4. a. Maintain normal activity levels.
   b. Maintain normal pulmonary function.
   c. Prevent chronic symptoms and recurrent exacerbations.
   d. Provide optimum drug therapy with minimum or no adverse effects.
   e. Assist the child in living as normal and happy a life as possible.
5. a. The parents will administer daily medications to prevent asthma symptoms.
   b. The parents and child will follow the daily asthma action plan.
   c. The family will remove allergens from the home.
6. Techniques aimed at the prevention and reduction of exposure to airborne allergens and irritants (eg, elimination of dust mites, cockroaches, tobacco smoke)

CHAPTER 22

Review of Essential Concepts

1. Any of the five responses are appropriate
   a. Fever
   b. Vomiting, diarrhea
   c. High-output kidney failure
   d. Diabetes insipidus
   e. Diabetic ketoacidosis
   f. Burns
   g. Shock
   h. Tachypnea
   i. Radiant warmer or phototherapy
   j. Postoperative bowel surgery

2. Compared with older children and adults, infants and young children have a greater fluid intake and output relative to size. Water and electrolyte disturbances occur more frequently and more rapidly in infants and children, who adjust less promptly to these alterations. The infant's relatively greater body surface area (BSA) allows larger quantities of fluid to be lost through the skin.
3. extracellular fluid, water loss
4. skin, respiratory tract
5. To support cellular and tissue growth
6. a. T
   b. F
   c. F. Rehydration may proceed by administering 2 to 5 ml of oral rehydration solution by syringe or small cup every 2 to 3 minutes.
   d. T
7. a. 4
   b. 2
   c. 3
   d. 1
8. A variety of viral, bacterial, and parasitic pathogens
9. Chronic
10. d
11. Rotavirus
12. glucose intolerance, fat malabsorption
13. a. Assessment of fluid and electrolyte imbalance
   b. Rehydration
   c. Maintenance fluid therapy
   d. Reintroduction of an adequate diet
14. a. Oral rehydration solution should be administered in small quantities at frequent intervals.
   b. Vomiting is not a contraindication to oral rehydration therapy unless it is severe.
   c. Introduction of the normal diet should be resumed when oral rehydration fluid is tolerated.
   d. Slightly higher stool output initially occurs with continuation of a normal diet.
15. prevention
16. F. Constipation is an alteration in the frequency, consistency, or ease of passing stool.

17. dietary practices, environmental changes or normal development
18. a. Restoring regular evacuation of stool
   b. Shrinking the distended rectum to its normal size
   c. Promoting regular toileting routine
19. Hirschsprung disease
20. anal stricture, incontinence
21. Vomiting
22. Detection and treatment of the cause of the vomiting and prevention of complications
23. The transfer of gastric contents into the esophagus
24. When complications such as failure to thrive, respiratory problems, or dysphagia develop
25. Recurrent abdominal pain is characterized by three or more separate episodes of abdominal pain at least 3 months before diagnosis that interferes with daily activities.
26. a. Periumbilical pain that may descend to the lower right quadrant
   b. Fever
   c. Rigid abdomen
   d. Decreased or absent bowel sounds
   e. Vomiting
   f. Constipation or diarrhea
   g. Anorexia
   h. Tachycardia; rapid, shallow breathing
   i. Pallor
   j. Lethargy
   k. Irritability
   l. Stooped posture
27. It is the most intense site of pain with appendicitis.
28. a. Bleeding
   b. Obstruction
   c. Inflammation
29. Surgical removal
30. Ulcerative colitis
31. ulcerative colitis
32. Crohn disease
33. gastric, duodenal
34. A, fecal-oral
35. a. parenterally
   b. percutaneously
   c. transmucosally
36. Hepatitis C
37. a. History
   b. Physical assessment
   c. Serologic markers in A, B, C
38. Proper handwashing and standard precautions

39. a. Infections
    b. Autoimmune disease
    c. Toxins
    d. Chronic diseases (eg, hemophilia and cystic fibrosis)
40. a. Monitoring liver function
    b. Managing specific complications such as esophageal varices and malnutrition
41. F
42. T
43. Feeding
44. a. Closure of the cleft
    b. Prevention of complications
    c. Facilitation of normal growth and development
45. a. Defective separation
    b. Incomplete fusion of the tracheal folds
    c. Altered cellular growth during embryonic development
46. A hernia that cannot be reduced easily is called an incarcerated hernia. A strangulated hernia is one in which the blood supply to the herniated organ is impaired.
47. paralytic ileus
48. nonbilious
49. Intussusception occurs when a proximal segment of the bowel telescopes into a more distal portion, pulling the mesentery with it.
50. 3 months and 3 years
51. F. Intussusception is more common in males.
52. Passage of normal brown stools
53. Malabsorption syndrome
54. a. Steatorrhea
    b. Exceedingly foul-smelling stools
    c. Malnutrition
    d. Muscle wasting
    e. Anemia
    f. Anorexia
    g. Abdominal distention
    h. Irritability
    i. Uncooperativeness
    j. Apathy
55. Celiac crisis
56. dietary management

Applying Critical Thinking to the Nursing Practice

A.
1. Fluid Volume Deficit related to excessive gastrointestinal losses in stool
2. a. Dry mucous membranes
   b. Decreased tears
   c. Irritability
   d. Slowed capillary refill (2 to 4 seconds)
   e. Normal to orthostatic blood pressure
   f. Weight loss 6% to 8%
   g. Slightly increased pulse rate
   h. Slight tachypnea
3. Kevin has signs of moderate dehydration, so 100 ml/kg of oral rehydration solution should be given plus an additional 10 mg/kg for each stool or vomitus.
4. Accurate measure of urinary output
5. The nurse should educate the parents about frequent and proper handwashing and the disposal of soiled diapers, clothes, and bed linens. The nurse should also stress the importance of maintaining certain "clean" areas and "dirty" areas, especially in the hospital, to keep diapers and other soiled articles away from clean areas, and by placing signs identifying "clean" (eg, bed, table) and "dirty" (eg, sink, bathroom) areas.

B.
1. The nurse tells the mother that no therapy is needed for an infant who is thriving and has no respiratory complications.
2. a. Elevate the head of the bed after feedings.
   b. Feedings thickened with 1 teaspoon to 1 tablespoon of rice cereal per ounce of formula might help alleviate the pain.
   c. Prone positioning may decrease episodes of gastroesophageal reflux, but all infants should sleep in the supine position due to the risk of sudden infant death syndrome.
3. Breastfeeding may continue, and the mother may provide more frequent feeding times or express the milk for thickening with rice cereal. The mother should avoid caffeine, chocolate, tobacco smoke, and alcohol when breastfeeding.

C.
1. Periumbilical pain
2. Fever, sudden relief from pain after perforation, subsequent increase in pain (usually diffuse and accompanied by rigid guarding of the abdomen), progressive abdominal distention, tachycardia, rapid shallow breathing, pallor, chills, irritability, and restlessness
3. Child's abdomen remains soft and nondistended; abdominal girth remains stable.

D.
1. Diarrhea, rectal bleeding, less frequent pain, moderate weight loss, mild rash, mild to moderate joint pain
2. When medical and nutritional therapies fail to prevent complications
3. Colorectal cancer

E.
1. a. Severity of hepatitis
   b. Medical management
   c. Factors influencing control and transmission of the disease
2. Consume a well-balanced diet and set a realistic schedule of rest and activity.

F.
1. In the first few weeks of life
2. Projectile nonbilious vomiting after a feeding. If the condition is not diagnosed early, dehydration, metabolic alkalosis, and failure to thrive may occur.
3. Feedings are usually instituted within 12 to 24 hours after surgery, beginning with clear liquids then advancing to formula or breast milk as tolerated. Observation and recording of feedings and the infant's responses to feedings are a vital part of postoperative care.

G.
1. The nurse must advise parents of the necessity of reading all label ingredients carefully to avoid hidden sources of gluten.
2. Wheat, rye, barley, oats
3. Corn, rice, and millet
4. Celiac Sprue Association

CHAPTER 23

Review of Essential Concepts
1. b
2. a
3. Echocardiography
4. a
5. increased oxygen concentration
6. c
7. a. 1
   b. 2
   c. 2
   d. 1

e. 1
f. 1
g. 2
8. a. 1
   b. 4
   c. 5
   d. 3
   e. 6
   f. 2
   g. 7
9. a. 1
   b. 1
   c. 2
   d. 2
   e. 2
   f. 2
10. d
11. a. 2
    b. 1
    c. 2
    d. 1
12. b
13. d
14. c
15. a
16. Any three of the following: nausea, vomiting, anorexia, bradycardia, dysrhythmias
17. a
18. a. F
    b. T
    c. F
    d. T
    e. F
    f. F
    g. T
    h. T
19. d
20. a. Assessing vital signs
    b. Assessing respiratory status
    c. Assessing rest and promoting activity
    d. Promoting comfort and providing emotional support
21. T
22. c
23. Rheumatic fever
24. c
25. a. Low-density lipoproteins contain low concentrations of triglycerides, high levels of cholesterol, and moderate levels of protein.
    b. High-density lipoproteins contain very low concentrations of triglycerides, relatively little cholesterol, and high levels of protein.
26. c
27. d

28. b
29. a
30. c
31. a
32. Orthotopic heart transplantation refers to removing the recipient's own heart and implanting a new heart from a donor who has had brain death but a healthy heart. The donor and recipient are matched by weight and blood type. Heterotopic heart transplantation refers to leaving the recipient's own heart in place and implanting a new heart to act as an additional pump or "piggyback" heart; this type of transplant is rarely done in children.
33. Secondary to a structural abnormality or an underlying pathologic process
34. Shock, circulatory failure
35. a. Hypovolemia
    b. Altered peripheral vascular resistance
    c. Pump failure
36. a. Ventilation
    b. Fluid administration
    c. Improvement of the heart's pumping action
37. The interaction of an allergen and a patient who is hypersensitive

Applying Critical Thinking to the Nursing Practice

A.
1. Height, weight, history of allergic reactions, signs and symptoms of infection, baseline oxygen saturation, signs of anxiety and/or fear, and location and marking of pedal pulses
2. a. To detect abnormalities in rate and rhythm; to identify a potential problem early
   b. To detect cardiac hemorrhage from perforation or bleeding at the site of the initial catheterization
   c. To detect vessel obstruction
   d. To detect possible arterial obstruction
3. Apply direct, continuous pressure 1 inch above the percutaneous skin site to localize pressure over the vessel puncture.

B.
1. Observing for signs of toxicity, calculating and administering the correct dosage, and instituting

parental teaching regarding the drug administration at home if needed
2. Because a pulse deficit, in which the radial pulse rate is lower than the apical, may be present with decreased cardiac output
3. Because the margin of safety between therapeutic, toxic, and lethal doses is very narrow

C.
1. a. Improves cardiac functioning by beneficial effects such as increased cardiac output, decreased heart size, decreased venous pressure, and relief of edema
   b. Removes accumulated fluid and sodium
2. Low potassium increases the cardiac effects of digitalis.
3. Decreased Cardiac Output related to structural defect, myocardial dysfunction
4. Any two of the following are acceptable:
   • Administer digoxin as ordered.
   • Make certain dosage is safe.
   • Check dosage with another nurse to ensure safety.
   • Count apical pulse for 1 full minute before giving medication.
   • Recognize signs of digoxin toxicity.
   • Ensure adequate intake of potassium.
   • Observe for signs of hypokalemia.
   • Monitor serum potassium levels, because a decrease enhances digoxin toxicity.
   • Check blood pressure.
   • Monitor electrolyte levels.
   • Attach cardiac monitor if ordered.
5. Heartbeat is strong, regular, and within normal limits for age, and peripheral perfusion is adequate.

D.
1. As soon as the diagnosis is suspected
2. Prevention. Parents need guidance to recognize the eventual hazards of continuing dependency and protectiveness as the child grows older, and the nurse can assist parents in learning ways to foster optimum development.

3. A clear explanation based on the parents' level of understanding; a review of the heart's basic structure and function; simple diagrams, pictures, or a model of the heart; written information about the specific condition; a glossary of frequently used terms; information about prognosis and treatment options
4. Recognize that more families are using the Internet as a source of information. It is important for parents to realize that not all websites offer accurate information.

E.
1. Anaphylaxis to strawberries
2. Because she is not exhibiting respiratory distress or cardiovascular compromise, antihistamines such as diphenhydramine (Benadryl) and epinephrine can be administered.
3. Ensuring adequate ventilation by establishing an airway, elevating the bed, preparing for the administration of oxygen, administering emergency medications, and preparing for the initiation of cardiopulmonary resuscitation

CHAPTER 24

Review of Essential Concepts
1. a. Child's lack of energy
   b. Food diary of poor sources of iron intake
   c. Frequent report of infections
   d. Bleeding that is difficult to control
2. shift to the left
3. Anemia
4. a. Etiology and physiology: manifested by erythrocyte or hemoglobin depletion
   b. Morphology: the characteristic changes in red blood cell size, shape, or color
5. T
6. a. 4
   b. 1
   c. 2
   d. 3
7. a. 4.5 to 5.5 million/mm^3; number of RBCs/mm^3 of blood
   b. 11.5 to 15.5 g/dl; amount of Hgb/g/dl of whole blood
   c. 35% to 45%; percentage or volume of packed RBCs to whole blood

   d. 4.5 to 13.5 × 10³ cells/mm^3; number of WBCs/mm^3 of blood
   e. 150 to 400 × 10³ cells/mm^3; number of platelets/mm^3 of blood
8. Primarily cow milk intake and not eating an adequate amount of iron-containing food
9. It should be given as prescribed in two divided doses between meals with citrus fruit or juice to increase absorption of the medication.
10. To reverse anemia by treating the underlying cause
11. a. Persistent bleeding
    b. Iron malabsorption
    c. Noncompliance
    d. Improper iron administration
    e. Other causes of anemia
12. 5, 6
13. circulatory overload
14. Stools turning a tarry green or black color, staining of teeth
15. a. Reinforce the importance of administering iron supplementation in the exclusively breastfed infant by 4 months of age since breast milk is a low iron source.
    b. Reinforce the importance of using iron-fortified formula and introducing iron-fortified cereal at 6 months of age.
16. Because iron ingestion in excessive quantities is toxic or even fatal
17. a. Obstruction caused by sickled RBCs
    b. Vascular inflammation
    c. Increased RBC destruction
18. Heterozygous persons who have both normal HbA and abnormal HbS
19. a. Vaso-occlusive crisis
    b. Sequestration crisis
    c. Aplastic crisis
    d. Hyperhemolytic crisis
20. Sickledex, Hgb electrophoresis
21. a. To prevent sickling phenomena, which are responsible for the pathologic sequelae
    b. To treat the medical emergencies of the sickle cell crisis
22. F. Oxygen administration is usually not effective in reversing sickling.
23. Prolonged oxygen administration
24. Acute chest syndrome

25. Repeat cerebrovascular accidents can cause progressively greater brain damage in untreated children.
26. a. 3
    b. 1
    c. 4
    d. 2
27. a. Small stature
    b. Delayed sexual maturation
    c. Bronzed, freckled complexion
28. To maintain sufficient hemoglobin B (Hgb) levels in order to prevent bone marrow expansion and the resulting bony deformities, and to provide sufficient RBCs to support normal growth and normal physical activity
29. Iron overload (hemosiderosis)
30. chelators
31. All fevers of 38.5° C (101.3° F) or higher
32. a. Anemia
    b. Leukopenia
    c. Decreased platelet count (thrombocytopenia)
33. bone marrow examination
34. Hemophilia
35. a. Factor VIII deficiency (hemophilia A or classic hemophilia)
    b. Factor IX deficiency (hemophilia B or Christmas disease)
36. a. Swelling
    b. Warmth
    c. Redness
    d. Severe pain with loss of movement
37. Replacement of the missing clotting factor
38. a. Subcutaneous route is substituted for intramuscular injections when possible.
    b. Venipunctures are used for blood sampling.
    c. Aspirin or aspirin-containing products should be used.
39. a. Factor replacement therapy according to the established medical protocol
    b. Supportive measures, such as RICE (rest, ice, compression, elevation)
40. a. Thrombocytopenia
    b. Absence or minimal signs of bleeding
    c. A normal bone marrow with normal or increased number of immature platelets and eosinophils

287

41. 20,000/mm^3, supportive
42. consumption coagulopathy
43. a. Diffuse fibrin deposition in the microvasculature
    b. Consumption of coagulation factors
    c. Endogenous generation of thrombin and plasmin
44. bleeding, clotting
45. Control of the underlying or initiating cause
46. lymphocytes, monocytes
47. a. Perinatal transmission (in utero, delivery, breastfeeding)
    b. Horizontal transmission (sexual contact or parenteral exposure to blood or body fluids with visible blood)
48. a. Lymphadenopathy
    b. Hepatosplenomegaly
    c. Oral candidiasis
    d. Chronic or recurrent diarrhea
    e. Failure to thrive
    f. Developmental delay
    g. Parotitis
49. a. HIV
    b. There is no cure. Therapy is directed primarily toward slowing growth of the virus; preventing and managing the opportunistic infections; providing nutritional support and symptomatic treatment; using antiviral drugs; providing prophylaxis for *Pneumocystis carinii* pneumonia with trimethoprim-sulfamethoxazole; providing prophylaxis for disseminated *Mycobacterium avium*-intracellulare complex, candidiasis, and herpes simplex; providing immunizations; and managing nutrition.
    c. It is changing from a fatal to a chronic disease.
50. Education should include the routes of transmission, the hazards of IV and other recreational drug use, and the value of sexual abstinence and safe sex practices.
51. humoral, cell-mediated
52. a. Chronic infections
    b. Failure to completely recover from infections
    c. Frequent reinfections
    d. Infection with unusual agents
53. Hematopoietic stem cell transplant
54. congenital X-linked

55. increased bleeding at the circumcision site, bloody diarrhea
56. a. Hemolytic reactions
    b. Febrile reactions
    c. Allergic reactions
    d. Circulatory overload
    e. Air emboli
    f. Hypothermia
    g. Electrolyte disturbances
57. Apheresis

Applying Critical Thinking to the Nursing Practice

A.
1. a. Explaining the significance of each test
   b. Encouraging parents or another supportive person to be with Regan during the procedure
   c. Allowing Regan to play with the equipment on a doll
2. Prematurity, consumption of cow's milk before 12 months of age, excessive cow's milk ingestion, age 12 to 36 months
3. Educate the family on an appropriate amount of cow's milk for their child, how cow's milk interferes with iron absorption, the proper administration of oral iron, and the introduction of solid foods (iron-fortified cereal) at an appropriate age.

B.
1. a. Pain related to tissue ischemia
   b. Altered Tissue Perfusion related to impaired arterial blood flow
2. Analyze the current drug dosage and suggest an increase to prevent, rather than treat, pain. Add psychologic support to counter depression, anxiety, and fear, if present. Opioids, such as immediate- and sustained-release morphine, oxycodone, hydromorphine, and methadone, can be given intravenously or orally. Administer medication around the clock or via patient-controlled analgesia.
3. Few, if any, children who receive opioids for severe pain become behaviorally addicted to the drug. When the pain is gone, the need for the drug is gone. Addiction is rare in children.

C.
1. a. Deficiency of factor VIII
   b. Subcutaneous and intramuscular hemorrhages

2. Replacement of the missing clotting factor
3. No. Venipunctures for blood samples are usually preferred for these children because there is usually less bleeding after the venipuncture than after a finger or heel stick.
4. Aerobic exercise, stretching exercises, swimming, walking, jogging, tennis, golf, fishing, bowling

D.
1. a. Review of standard precautions describing proper management of blood and body fluids
   b. Safety issues, such as the storage of medications and medical equipment
   c. Dan's parents have the legal right to decide whether they inform daycare employees of their child's diagnosis
2. Immunizations are recommended for all children infected with HIV. Varicella and measles-mumps-rubella vaccines can be administered only if there is no evidence of severe immunocompromise.
3. Any three of the following are acceptable:
   • Risk for Infection related to impaired body defenses, presence of infective organisms
   • Altered Nutrition: Less Than Body Requirements related to recurrent illness, diarrheal losses, loss of appetite, oral candidiasis
   • Impaired Social Interaction related to physical limitations, hospitalizations, social stigma toward HIV infection
   • Chronic Pain related to disease process
   • Interrupted Family Processes related to having an infant with a dreaded and life-threatening disease

CHAPTER 25

Review of Essential Concepts
1. a. Chromosome abnormalities
   b. Genetic syndromes
   c. Immunodeficiencies
2. T
3. T

4. a. Use of multimodal therapy
   b. Enrollment of large numbers of children in cooperative group clinical trials or protocols
   c. Improvements in supportive care
5. primary mechanism of action
6. anaphylaxis; urticaria, angioedema, flushing, rashes, difficulty breathing, hypotension, and nausea/vomiting
7. By therapeutically changing the host's biologic response to tumor cells
8. a. Children who have diseases that require high doses of chemotherapy
   b. Children who have diseases that require replacement of dysfunctional bone marrow
9. F. The hallmark metabolic abnormalities of tumor lysis syndrome include hyperuricemia, hypocalcemia, hyperphosphatemia, and hyperkalemia.
10. a. High white blood cell count at diagnosis
    b. Large tumor burden
    c. Sensitivity to chemotherapy
    d. High proliferative rate
11. Hyperleukocytosis
12. superior vena cava syndrome, airway, respiratory
13. Back pain
14. a. Overwhelming infection
    b. General malaise
    c. Invasion of organisms producing secondary infections
15. Colony stimulating factors
16. Judicious administration of platelet concentrates or platelet-rich plasma
17. Activities that might cause injury or bleeding, such as riding bicycles or skateboards, roller skating or in-line skating, climbing trees or playground equipment, and contact sports such as football or soccer
18. packed red blood cells
19. Administration of an antiemetic before the chemotherapy begins and regular administration for at least 24 hours after chemotherapy
20. Oral supplements with high-protein and high-calorie foods; using whole milk, adding tofu (high in protein) to most meals, and serving full-fat instead of nonfat or low-fat items; cooking with butter; putting sugar or cheese on foods; and making high-calorie snacks such as trail mix, peanut butter, or dried fruit readily available for the child
21. F. Lemon glycerin swabs should not be used in children with oral ulcers because of the drying effects on the mucosa.
22. T
23. Severe constipation
24. Post-irritation somnolence, 4 to 15 days
25. a. Liberal oral or parenteral fluid intake
    b. Frequent voiding immediately after feeling the urge
    c. Administration of the drug early in the day
    d. Administration of mesna
26. a. Child can wear a disposable surgical cap to collect the shed hair
    b. The hair can be cut short or shaved
27. Because of the aggressive preconditioning therapy used to remove the marrow and the potential for complications while waiting for engraftment of transplanted stem cells
28. T
29. F. The child receiving chemotherapy for cancer should not receive live, attenuated vaccines.
30. a. Varicella-zoster immune globulin
    b. Antiviral agent such as acyclovir
31. Medication schedules, observing for side effects or toxicities that require further evaluation, taking measures to prevent or manage these problems, and caring for special devices such as central venous catheters
32. a. Acute lymphoid leukemia
    b. Acute myelogenous leukemia
33. immature white blood cells
34. a. Anemia from decreased erythrocytes
    b. Infection from neutropenia
    c. Bleeding from decreased platelet production
35. Initial white blood cell count, patient's age at diagnosis, cytogenetics, immunologic subtype, and the child's sex
36. Bone marrow aspiration or biopsy
37. a. Induction therapy
    b. Intensification or consolidation therapy
    c. Maintenance therapy
38. 5%
39. Children with leukemia are at risk for invasion of the central nervous system by the leukemic cells.
40. a. Hodgkin disease originates in the lymphoid system and primarily involves the lymph nodes. It predictably metastasizes to nonnodal or extra-lymphatic sites, especially the spleen, liver, bone marrow, and lungs.
    b. Non-Hodgkin lymphoma is usually diffuse, rather than nodular; the cell type is evenly split between B-cell and T-cell lineages; and dissemination occurs early, more often than in Hodgkin disease, and rapidly.
41. Enlarged, firm, nontender, movable nodes in the supraclavicular or cervical area
42. a. Anatomic location
    b. Size
43. Removal of the tumor without residual neurologic damage
44. Sluggish, dilated, or unequal pupils
45. Because of hyperthermia resulting from surgical intervention in the hypothalamus or brainstem and from some types of general anesthesia
46. Neuroblastoma
47. a. 3
    b. 2
    c. 4
    d. 5
    e. 1
48. 15 years, males
49. a. Ewing sarcoma most commonly involves the pelvis, long bones of the lower extremities, and chest wall.
    b. Osteosarcoma lesions are most commonly located in the metaphyseal region of the bone, often involving the long bones.
50. prosthesis
51. This symptom is characterized by sensations such as tingling,

289

itching, and, more frequently, pain felt in the amputated limb.
52. Radiotherapy and chemotherapy
53. Painless swelling or mass within the abdomen and a firm, non-tender mass confined to one side deep within the flank
54. Manipulation of the mass may cause dissemination of cancer cells to adjacent and distant sites
55. a. Careful assessment for signs of the tumor, especially during well-child examinations
    b. Preparation of the child and family for the multiple diagnostic tests
    c. Supportive care during each stage of multimodal therapy
56. Retinoblastoma

Applying Critical Thinking to the Nursing Practice

A.
1. Patient will experience minimized risk of infection.
2. a. Place child in a private room to minimize exposure to infective organisms.
   b. Screen all visitors and staff for signs of infection.
   c. Monitor the child's temperature to detect possible infection.
   d. Administer antibiotics as prescribed.

B.
1. Blood pressure monitor, oxygen with a bag and valve mask, and suction
2. a. Hypersensitivity reaction or anaphylaxis
   b. The nurse discontinues the drug, flushes and maintains the intravenous line with saline, and monitors Janet's vital signs and subsequent responses.

C.
1. Pupillary reaction to light, level of consciousness, sleep patterns, response to stimuli, and steady increase in alertness
2. Every precaution is used to prevent jarring or misalignment to prevent undue strain on the sutures. Two nurses, one supporting the head and the other the body, are needed. The use of a turning sheet may facilitate turning a heavy child.

3. Providing a quiet, dimly lit environment; restricting visitors; preventing any sudden jarring movement, such as banging into the bed; preventing an increase in intracranial pressure; administration of opioids, acetaminophen, or codeine as prescribed
4. "The surgeon removed most of the tumor, and the rest will be treated with special drugs and x-ray treatments."

D.
1. Straightforward honesty is essential; if Katie desires more information, it may be helpful to introduce her to another amputee before surgery or to show her pictures of a prosthesis; answer questions without offering additional information.
2. Katie needs to know that the sensations are real, not imagined. Various medications, such as morphine, gabapentin, and ketamine can be used for phantom limb pain.

CHAPTER 26

Review of Essential Concepts

1. d
2. urinalysis
3. a. 4
   b. 2
   c. 1
   d. 5
   e. 3
   f. 6
4. b
5. a
6. a. Eliminate current infection.
   b. Identify contributing factors to reduce the risk for recurrence.
   c. Prevent systemic spread of the infection.
   d. Preserve renal function.
7. F. Reflux increases the chance for febrile urinary tract infection but does not cause it.
8. a. High fevers
   b. Vomiting
   c. Chills
9. a. T
   b. T
10. a. F
    b. T
    c. T
    d. F
11. c

12. b
13. a. Reduce excretion of urinary protein.
    b. Reduce fluid retention in the tissues.
    c. Prevent infection.
    d. Minimize complications related to therapies.
14. a. Weight gain
    b. Rounded moon face
    c. Behavior changes
    d. Increased appetite
15. d
16. F. Moderate sodium restriction and even fluid restriction may be instituted for children with hypertension and edema.
17. c
18. b
19. a. Early diagnosis
    b. Supportive care
20. a. The accumulation of nitrogenous waste within the blood
    b. A more advanced condition than azotemia in which retention of nitrogenous products produces toxic symptoms
21. c
22. d
23. a
24. b
25. d
26. a. Peritoneal dialysis
    b. Hemodialysis
    c. Hemofiltration
27. d
28. b
29. F
30. transplantation

Applying Critical Thinking to the Nursing Practice

A.
1. a. Fever
   b. Poor appetite
   c. Excessive thirst
   d. Incontinence
   e. Painful urination
2. a. Eliminate current infection.
   b. Identify contributing factors to decrease the risk of recurrence.
   c. Prevent systemic spread of infection.
   d. Preserve renal function.
3. The decision is based on the proper identification of the pathogen, the child's history of antibiotic use, and the location of the infection.
4. Prevention of recurrence

B.

1. Nephrotic syndrome
2. Fluid Volume Excess
3. The presence of edema may predispose the child to skin breakdown and may make routine care more difficult.
4. Upper respiratory tract infection

C.

1. Hemolytic uremic syndrome
2. Hemodialysis or peritoneal dialysis
3. a. The disease, its implications, and the therapeutic plan
   b. The possible psychologic effects of the disease and its treatment
   c. The technical aspects of the procedure
4. Tina will consume a healthy diet.
5. The nurse could observe Tina and her family successfully coping with the stresses of illness (eg, performing routine care of the activities of daily living).

D.

1. Patient will maintain near-normal electrolyte levels.
2. a. Assist with dialysis to maintain excretory function.
   b. Administer sodium polystyrene sulfate (Kayexalate) as prescribed to decrease serum potassium levels.
   c. Provide a diet low in potassium, sodium, and phosphorus.
   d. Observe for evidence of accumulated waste products (hyperkalemia, hyperphosphatemia, uremia).

CHAPTER 27

Review of Essential Concepts

1. spontaneous, elicited reflex, primitive reflexes
2. a. Family history
   b. Health history
   c. Physical evaluation of infants
3. a. Tense, bulging fontanel; separated cranial sutures; Macewen sign; irritability; drowsiness; high-pitched cry; increased occipital frontal circumference; distended scalp veins; poor feeding; crying when disturbed; "setting sun" sign
   b. Headache, nausea, forceful vomiting, diplopia, seizures, drowsiness, decline in school performance, diminished physical activity and motor performance, increased sleeping, inability to follow commands, lethargy
4. Bradycardia, decreased motor response to commands, decreased sensory response to painful stimuli, alterations in pupil size and reactivity, extension or flexion posturing, Cheyne-Stokes respiration, papilledema, decreased consciousness, coma
5. a. Alertness: an aroused or waking state that includes the ability to respond to stimuli
   b. Cognitive power: the ability to process stimuli and produce verbal and motor responses
6. Coma
7. a. 3
   b. 8
   c. 1
   d. 5
   e. 2
   f. 7
   g. 6
   h. 4
8. a. Eye opening
   b. Verbal response
   c. Motor response
9. This allows for comparison of the findings so the observer can detect subtle changes in the neurologic status that might not otherwise be evident.
10. The sudden appearance of a fixed and dilated pupil(s)
11. 24 to 48 hours after injury
12. a. Flexion posturing is seen with severe dysfunction of the cerebral cortex or with lesions to corticospinal tracts above the brainstem. Typical flexion posturing includes rigid flexion, with arms held tightly to the body; flexed elbows, wrists, and fingers; plantar-flexed feet; legs extended and internally rotated; and possibly the presence of fine tremors or intense stiffness.
    b. Extension posturing is a sign of dysfunction at the level of the midbrain or lesions to the brainstem. It is characterized by rigid extension and pronation of the arms and legs, flexed wrists and fingers, clenched jaw, extended neck, and possibly an arched back.
13. Moro, tonic neck, withdrawal
14. Chloral hydrate, benzodiazepines
15. a. Ensuring a patent airway, breathing, and circulation
    b. Stabilizing the spine
    c. Treating shock
    d. Reducing intracranial pressure if present
16. Changes in behavior (eg, increased agitation or rigidity) and alterations in vital signs (eg, increased heart rate, respiratory rate, and blood pressure, and decreased oxygen saturation)
17. a. Glasgow Coma Scale evaluation of less than or equal to 8
    b. Glasgow Coma Scale evaluation greater than 8 with respiratory assistance
    c. Deterioration of condition
    d. Subjective judgment regarding clinical appearance and response
18. a. T
    b. F. The head of an infant and toddler is the most likely body part to be injured.
    c. T
19. Confusion and amnesia
20. Contusions are used to describe visible bruising and tearing of cerebral tissue. Contusions represent petechial hemorrhages or localized bruising along the superficial aspects of the brain.
21. a. F. The lower incidence of epidural hematoma in childhood has been attributed to the fact that the middle meningeal artery is not embedded in the bone surface of the skull until approximately 2 years of age.
    b. T
    c. T
    d. F. These are signs of brainstem involvement.
    e. T
    f. T
22. The most important nursing observation is assessment of the child's level of consciousness.
23. a. 4
    b. 3
    c. 1
    d. 2
24. a. Hypoxia

b. Aspiration
c. Hypothermia
25. Resuscitative measures including maximum ventilatory and circulatory support
26. meningitis, encephalitis
27. *Haemophilus influenzae, Streptococcus pneumoniae*
28. a. Group b streptococci
    b. *S. pneumoniae*
    c. *N. meningitidis*
29. a. T
    b. F. It is less common than invasion from an infection elsewhere in the body.
    c. F
    d. T
30. Because he or she may have (overwhelming) meningococcemia.
31. a. Isolation precautions
    b. Initiation of antimicrobial therapy
    c. Maintenance of hydration
    d. Maintenance of ventilation
    e. Reduction of increased intracranial pressure
    f. Management of systemic shock
    g. Control of seizures
    h. Control of temperature
    i. Treatment of complications
32. a. Direct invasion of the central nervous system (CNS) by a virus
    b. Postinfectious involvement of the CNS after a viral disease
33. supportive
34. a. The child's age
    b. The type of organism
    c. Residual neurologic damage
35. Rabies
36. a. Thorough cleansing of the wound with soap and water
    b. Administration of rabies vaccine
    c. Administration of rabies immunoglobulin
37. metabolic encephalopathy
38. a. Fever
    b. Profoundly impaired consciousness
    c. Disordered hepatic function
39. aspirin
40. liver biopsy
41. type, etiology
42. Epilepsy is defined as two or more unprovoked seizures more than 24 hours apart and can be caused by a variety of pathologic processes in the brain.

43. a. Partial seizures, which have a local onset and involve a relatively small location in the brain
    b. Generalized seizures, which involve both hemispheres of the brain from onset or secondarily generalize from partial seizures
44. a. Sudden excessive excitation
    b. Loss of inhibition within the neuronal circuits
45. a. Staring and migraine headaches
    b. Toxic effects of drugs
    c. Syncope (fainting)
    d. Breath-holding spells in infants and young children
    e. Movement disorders (tics, tremor, chorea)
    f. Prolonged QT syndrome
    g. Sleep disturbances (night terrors)
    h. Psychogenic seizures
    i. Rage attacks
    j. Transient ischemic attacks (rare in children)
46. Electroencephalography; It confirms the presence of abnormal electrical discharges and provides information on the seizure type and the focus.
47. a. Control the seizures or reduce their frequency.
    b. Discover and correct the cause of seizures when possible
48. The administration of the appropriate antiepileptic drug, or combination of drugs, in a dosage that provides the desired effect without causing undesirable side effects or toxic reactions
49. Treatment is begun with a single drug known to be effective for the child's seizure type that has the lowest risk of adverse side effects. The dosage is gradually increased until the seizures are controlled or the maximum recommended dose has been reached.
50. The drugs should be reduced gradually over weeks or months.
51. ketogenic
52. surgical removal
53. Status epilepticus
54. Only about half of children who experience a first seizure will experience additional seizures.

55. vitamin D, folic acid
56. Keeping side rails raised when the child is sleeping or resting, keeping side rails and other hard objects padded, using a waterproof mattress or pad on the bed or crib, using appropriate precautions during potentially hazardous activities, having the child carry or wear medical identification, alerting other caregivers to the need for any special precautions, child may not drive or operate hazardous machinery or equipment unless seizure-free for a designated period of time
57. Febrile
58. Hydrocephalus
59. a. Impaired absorption of cerebrospinal fluid (CSF) within the subarachnoid space (communicating)
    b. Obstruction to the flow of CSF within the ventricles (noncommunicating)
60. myelomeningocele
61. a. Abnormally rapid head growth
    b. Bulging fontanels
    c. Anterior fontanel is tense, bulging, and nonpulsatile
    d. Dilated scalp veins
    e. Separated sutures
    f. Macewen sign on percussion
    g. Thinning of skull bones
    h. Frontal enlargement or "bossing"
    i. Depressed eyes ("setting sun" sign)
    j. Sluggish pupils with unequal response to light
62. Surgical placement of a shunt to drain the cerebrospinal fluid

Applying Critical Thinking to the Nursing Practice

A.
1. Risk for Ineffective Cerebral Tissue Perfusion, related to head injury, secondary to intracranial pressure
2. A neurosurgical emergency

B.
1. a. Increased agitation
   b. Increased rigidity
   c. Increased heart rate
   d. Increased respiratory rate
   e. Increased blood pressure
   f. Decreased oxygen saturation
2. a. Assess for evidence of pain.

b. Use the pain assessment record to document the effectiveness of interventions.
c. Administer pain medication as needed.
3. a. Vital signs
b. Pupillary reactions
c. Level of consciousness
4. Administration of artificial tears (methylcellulose) and eye patches
C.
1. Rhinorrhea; cerebrospinal fluid from a skull fracture
2. a. Hypoxia
b. Aspiration
c. Hypothermia
D.
1. Clinical manifestations include fever, poor feeding, vomiting, marked irritability, seizures, a high-pitched cry, and a bulging fontanel. Nuchal rigidity may or may not be present. Brudzinski and Kernig signs are not usually used in making the diagnosis, since they are difficult to evaluate in children in this age group.
2. Administer the antibiotic as soon as it is ordered.
E.
1. a. Ascertain the type of seizure the child has experienced.
b. Attempt to understand the cause of the events.
2. a. Do not attempt to restrain him or use force.
b. Remove objects from the bed.
c. Place a folded blanket under his head.
d. Protect him from injury on side rails.
e. Have someone in the room with him at all times.
f. Make certain he calls for assistance when getting out of bed.
F.
1. a. Abnormally rapid head growth
b. Bulging fontanels
c. Dilated scalp veins
d. Separated sutures
e. Macewen sign
f. Thinning of the skull bones
2. a. Position Adam on his unoperated side to prevent pressure on the shunt valve.
b. Keep Adam flat to prevent too-rapid reduction of intracranial fluid.

c. Manage pain with acetaminophen, acetaminophen with codeine, or opioids.
d. Monitor his neurologic status.
e. Monitor his vital signs.
f. Observe for abdominal distention.
g. Monitor his hydration status.
h. Monitor for infection at the operative site.
i. Inspect the incision site for leakage.
j. Provide meticulous skin care.
3. Family discusses their feelings and concerns regarding the child's condition; family demonstrates adequate and proper care of Adam in relation to his diagnosis and the treatment of hydrocephalus.

CHAPTER 28

Review of Essential Concepts

1. c
2. d
3. b
4. Because these children frequently have parents who experienced similar slow growth patterns and delayed sexual maturation.
5. Replacement of growth hormone
6. At night
7. a
8. Early identification of children with excessive growth rates
9. Manifestations of sexual development before age 9 years in boys or age 8 years in girls
10. diabetes insipidus, diuresis
11. a. Polyuria
b. Polydipsia
12. Hormone replacement
13. Oversecretion of the posterior pituitary hormone or antidiuretic hormone
14. Fluid restriction
15. b
16. It regulates the basal metabolic rate and thereby controls the processes of growth and tissue differentiation.
17. hypothyroidism
18. goiter
19. Lymphocytic thyroiditis, juvenile autoimmune thyroiditis
20. b
21. a. Irritability
b. Hyperactivity

c. Short attention span
d. Tremors
e. Insomnia
f. Emotional lability
22. a. Antithyroid drugs, which interfere with the biosynthesis of thyroid hormone, including propylthiouracil (PTU) and methimazole (MTZ, Tapazole)
b. Subtotal thyroidectomy
c. Ablation with radioiodine (131I iodide)
23. agranulocytosis (severe leukopenia)
24. d
25. serum calcium, serum phosphorus
26. a. Acute adrenocortical insufficiency
b. Hyperfunction of the adrenal gland
27. Monitor and observe for signs of hypokalemia or hyperkalemia (eg, weakness, poor muscle control, paralysis, cardiac dysrhythmias, and apnea).
28. cortisol
29. moon
30. genotype, cortisone
31. Injectable hydrocortisone
32. Increased production of catecholamines
33. insulin
34. glucose
35. a. Type 1 diabetes mellitus (DM) is characterized by destruction of the pancreatic cells, which produce insulin; this usually leads to absolute insulin deficiency. Type 1 DM has two forms. Immune-mediated DM results from an autoimmune destruction of the cells; it typically starts in children or young adults who are slim, but it can arise in adults of any age. Idiopathic type 1 refers to rare forms of the disease that have no known cause.
b. Type 2 DM arises because of insulin resistance, in which the body fails to use insulin properly, combined with relative (rather than absolute) insulin deficiency. People with type 2 can range from being predominantly insulin-resistant with relative insulin

deficiency to being predominantly deficient in insulin secretion with some insulin resistance. It typically occurs in those who are over 45 years of age, are overweight and sedentary, and have a family history of diabetes.

36. a. T
    b. F
    c. T
    d. T
    e. T
    f. F
    g. T
    h. F
37. a
38. b
39. a. Polyphagia
    b. Polydipsia
    c. Polyuria
40. 126 mg/dl, 200 mg/dl, 200 mg/dl
41. a. 3
    b. 2
    c. 1
    d. 4
42. a. 2
    b. 1
    c. 3
43. Insulin pumps
44. Self-monitoring of blood glucose
45. Lowers blood glucose levels
46. The Somogyi effect may occur at any time but often entails an elevated blood glucose level at bedtime and a drop at 2 am, with a rebound rise following. The treatment for this phenomenon is decreasing the nocturnal insulin dose to prevent the 2 am hypoglycemia. The rebound rise in the blood glucose level is a result of counterregulatory hormones (epinephrine, growth hormone, and corticosteroids), which are stimulated by hypoglycemia.
47. Insulin reactions; bursts of physical activity without additional food; or delayed, omitted, or incompletely consumed meals
48. c
49. glucose (ie, sugar)
50. venous access

Applying Critical Thinking to the Nursing Practice

A.
1. a. Polyuria
   b. Polydipsia

2. a. Overgrowth of long bones; may reach a height of 8 feet
   b. Rapid and increased development of muscles and viscera
   c. Weight increase, but in proportion to height
   d. Proportional enlargement of head circumference
3. a. Enlarged thyroid gland
   b. Tracheal compression
   c. Hyperthyroidism
4. a. Severe irritability
   b. Restlessness
   c. Vomiting
   d. Diarrhea
   e. Hyperthermia
   f. Hypertension
   g. Severe tachycardia
   h. Prostration
5. a.

B.
1. Chronic adrenocortical insufficiency
2. They must demonstrate awareness of the continuous need for cortisol replacement. Sudden termination of the drug places the child in danger of an acute adrenal crisis.
3. Weakness, poor muscle control, paralysis, cardiac dysrhythmias, and apnea

C.
1. Any five of the following are acceptable:
   • Hypertension
   • Tachycardia
   • Headache
   • Decreased gastrointestinal activity, constipation
   • Anorexia
   • Weight loss
   • Hyperglycemia
   • Polyuria
   • Polydipsia
   • Hyperventilation
   • Nervousness
   • Heat intolerance
   • Diaphoresis
   • Signs of congestive heart failure in severe cases
2. catecholamines; stimulate severe hypertension and tachyarrhythmias

D.
1. Ketoacidosis
2. Insulin replacement therapy
3. Insulin pump, because he will only need to insert the needle into his subcutaneous tissue every

48 hours, instead of several times a day with self-injections
4. Blood glucose monitoring
5. Education
6. a. Hypoglycemia
   b. Immediate treatment of hypoglycemia
7. a. He will recognize signs of hypoglycemia early and be particularly alert at times when blood glucose levels are lowest (after or during physical activity without additional food).
   b. Offer 10 to 15 g of readily absorbed carbohydrates, such as orange juice, hard candy, or milk, to elevate the blood glucose level and alleviate symptoms of hypoglycemia.
   c. Follow with a complex carbohydrate and protein, such as bread or cracker spread with peanut butter or cheese, to maintain blood glucose level.
8. Child ingests an appropriate carbohydrate; child displays no evidence of hypoglycemia.
9. Being sick will increase his insulin needs. The nurse should stress the importance of giving insulin on time and the strong possibility that insulin doses typically need to be increased during sickness. It is also important that the nurse educates the parents of the importance of frequent blood glucose monitoring during illness.

CHAPTER 29

Review of Essential Concepts

1. a. Decreased muscle strength and mass
   b. Decreased metabolism
   c. Bone demineralization
2. When the arrangement of collagen, the main structural protein of connective tissues, is altered, resulting in a denser tissue that does not glide as easily. Eventually, muscles, tendons, and ligaments can shorten and reduce joint movement, ultimately producing contractures that restrict function.
3. a. Prolonged immobilization
   b. Mechanical ventilation

c. Orthotic and prosthetic devices, including wheelchairs and casts

4. a. Damage to the soft tissue, subcutaneous structures, and muscle
   b. Occurs when the force of stress on the ligament is so great that it displaces the normal position of the opposing bone ends or the bone end to its socket
   c. Occurs when trauma to a joint is so severe that a ligament is partially or completely torn or stretched by the force created as a joint is twisted or wrenched, often accompanied by damage to associated blood vessels, muscles, tendons, and nerves
   d. Microscopic tear to the musculotendinous unit; has features in common with sprains

5. a. Rest, Ice, Compression, Elevation
   b. Ice, Compression, Elevation, Support

6. osteogenesis imperfecta

7. simple, closed, open, compound

8. Radiographic examination

9. T

10. F. Spica casts immobilize the hip and knee.

11. a. To regain alignment and length of the bony fragments (reduction)
    b. To retain alignment and length (immobilization)
    c. To restore function to the injured parts
    d. To prevent further injury and deformity

12. a. Pain
    b. Pallor
    c. Pulselessness
    d. Paresthesia
    e. Paralysis
    f. Pressure

13. The extremity may continue to swell to the extent that the cast becomes a tourniquet, shutting off circulation and producing neurovascular complications. To prevent this, the body part can be elevated, thereby increasing venous return.

14. a. Traction is used to reduce or realign a fracture site; traction (forward force) is produced by attaching weight to the distal bone fragment.
    b. Countertraction is where the body weight provides backward force.
    c. Frictional force is the patient's contact with the bed.

15. a. The child's age
    b. The condition of the soft tissues
    c. The type and degree of displacement of the fracture

16. Distraction

17. A severed part should be rinsed with normal saline; wrapped loosely in sterile gauze and placed in a watertight plastic bag; cool the bag, without freezing, in ice water (do not pack in ice); label the bag with the patient's name, date, and time; and transport with the patient to the hospital.

18. a. Physiologic factors, which include maternal hormone secretion and intrauterine positioning
    b. Mechanical factors, which include breech presentation, multiple fetuses, oligohydramnios, large infant size, and continued maintenance of the hips in adduction and extension that will in time cause a dislocation
    c. Genetic factors, which entail a higher incidence of developmental dysplasia of the hip in siblings of affected infants and an even greater incidence of recurrence if a sibling and one parent were affected

19. Because ossification of the femoral head does not normally take place until the fourth to sixth month of life.

20. a. 5
    b. 2
    c. 3
    d. 4
    e. 1

21. a. correction of the deformity.
    b. maintenance of the correction until normal muscle balance is regained.
    c. follow-up observation to avert possible recurrence of the deformity.

22. chorionic villus sampling

23. fractures, bone deformity

24. a. positional contractures and deformities
    b. muscle weakness and osteoporosis
    c. malalignment of lower extremity joints prohibiting weight bearing

25. A disturbance of circulation to the femoral capital epiphysis producing an ischemic aseptic necrosis of the femoral head

26. a. Eliminate hip irritability.
    b. Restore and maintain adequate range of hip motion.
    c. Prevent capital femoral epiphyseal collapse, extrusion, or subluxation.
    d. Ensure a well-rounded femoral head at the time of healing.

27. Slipped capital femoral epiphysis

28. a. 2
    b. 1
    c. 3

29. By radiographs of the child in the standing position and use of the Cobb technique (standard measurement of angle curvature), which establishes the degree of curvature

30. a. Observation with regular clinical and radiographic evaluation
    b. Bracing and exercise
    c. Surgery

31. Curves greater than 45 degrees, progressive curves that do not respond to bracing, and progressive congenital and neuromuscular curves

32. Osteomyelitis, *Staphylococcus aureus*

33. Leukocytosis, elevated erythrocyte sedimentation rate, and C-reactive protein

34. intravenous, antibiotic

35. Physical therapy

36. Juvenile idiopathic arthritis; the name was changed in part because the term rheumatoid is only minimally applicable to this disease, since only a small percentage of children have a positive rheumatoid factor. Rheumatoid may also burden the family with images of adult disfiguring rheumatoid arthritis. Furthermore, the junior rheumatoid arthritis classification system focused more on disease at onset as opposed to disease

progression, which is more important.
37. a. To control pain
    b. To preserve joint range of motion and function
    c. To minimize the effects of inflammation, such as joint deformity
    d. To promote normal growth and development
38. a. Nonsteroidal antiinflammatory drugs
    b. Methotrexate
    c. Corticosteroids
    d. Biologic agents
39. T
40. F. Nonsteroidal antiinflammatory drugs are the first drugs used.
41. T
42. Systemic lupus erythematosus
43. Erythematous butterfly rash extending across the nose and cheeks, discolored rash, photosensitivity, mucocutaneous ulceration, alopecia, periungual telangiectasias
44. Corticosteroids
45. disease exacerbation, medication therapy

Applying Critical Thinking to the Nursing Practice

A.
1. Significant decrease in muscle size, strength, and endurance; bone demineralization, leading to osteoporosis; and contractures and decreased joint mobility
2. To prevent dependent edema and to stimulate circulation, respiratory function, gastrointestinal motility, and neurologic sensations
3. Decreased efficiency of orthostatic neurovascular reflexes, diminished vasopressor mechanism, altered distribution of blood volume, venous stasis, and dependent edema

B.
1. Subluxation or partial dislocation of the radial head (ie, nursemaid's elbow)
2. The practitioner manipulates the arm by applying firm finger pressure to the head of the radius, then supinates and flexes the forearm to return the bone structure to normal alignment. A

click may be heard or felt, and functional use of the arm returns within minutes.

C.
1. Any four of the following are acceptable:
Provide an alternating-pressure mattress underneath the hips and back.
Make total-body skin checks for redness or breakdown, especially over areas that receive the greatest pressures.
Wash and dry the skin daily.
Inspect pressure points daily or more if risk for breakdown is observed.
Use a skin breakdown assessment scale.
Stimulate circulation with gentle massage over the pressure areas.
Change position at least every 2 hours to relieve pressure.
Encourage increased intake of oral fluids.
Provide and encourage the patient to eat a balanced diet with fruits and vegetables.
2. a. Observe for correct body alignment.
   b. Check alignment after the child has moved.
   c. Maintain the correct angles at joints.

D.
1. a. Leg shortening on the affected side
   b. Asymmetry of the thigh and gluteal fold
   c. Limited abduction of the hip on the affected side
   d. Positive Ortolani test
   e. Positive Barlow test
2. Newborn infants who are tightly wrapped in blankets or other swaddling material or are strapped to cradle boards have the highest incidence of dislocation. In cultures such as Asia, where mothers traditionally carry infants on their backs or hips in the widely abducted straddle position, the disorder is virtually unknown.
3. By dynamic splinting in a safe position, with the proximal femur centered in the acetabulum in an attitude of flexion by a harness like the Pavlik harness

E.
1. Bone fragility, deformity, and fracture; blue sclerae; hearing

loss; and dentinogenesis imperfecta
2. a. Muscle weakness
   b. Osteoporosis

F.
1. Nonsteroidal antiinflammatory drugs; fewer side effects, easier to administer, and very effective
2. It is a diagnosis of exclusion based on the clinical criteria of age of onset before 16 years, arthritis in one or more joints for 6 weeks or longer, and exclusion of other conditions. Plain radiographs during initial imaging may show soft-tissue swelling and joint space widening from increased synovial fluid in the joint. Later films may show osteoporosis, narrow joint space, erosions, subluxation, and ankylosis.
3. a. Relieve pain.
   b. Promote general health.
   c. Facilitate compliance.
   d. Encourage health and exercise.
   e. Support the child and family in self-care, school participation, and recreational activities.

CHAPTER 30

Review of Essential Concepts

1. d
2. chorioamnionitis
3. a. Spastic cerebral palsy
   b. Dyskinetic cerebral palsy (nonspastic)
   c. Ataxic cerebral palsy (nonspastic)
   d. Mixed-type cerebral palsy (spastic cerebral palsy and dyskinetic cerebral palsy)
4. d
5. c
6. b
7. Botulinum toxin type A (Botox)
8. a. Constipation caused by neurologic deficits and lack of exercise
   b. Poor bladder control and urinary retention
   c. Chronic respiratory tract infections and aspiration pneumonia, which occur as a result of gastroesophageal reflux, abnormal muscle tone, immobility, and altered positioning

d. Skin problems as a result of altered positioning, poor nutrition, and immobility

e. Dental problems

9. d
10. a
11. a
12. c
13. a. Wheezing
    b. Facial swelling
    c. Facial rash
    d. Anaphylaxis
    e. Urticaria
14. a. Prevention of latex allergy
    b. Identification of children with a known hypersensitivity
15. Werdnig-Hoffmann
16. Symptomatically and preventively, primarily by preventing joint contractures and treating orthopedic problems, the most serious of which is scoliosis. Hip subluxation and dislocation may also occur.
17. Duchenne
18. Respiratory or cardiac failure
19. d
20. It is an acute demyelinating polyneuropathy with a progressive, usually ascending, flaccid paralysis.
21. Any three of the following
    a. Muscle tenderness
    b. Paresthesia and cramps
    c. Proximal symmetric muscle weakness
    d. Ascending paralysis from lower extremities
    e. Frequent involvement of muscles of trunk, upper extremities, and those supplied by cranial nerves (especially facial nerve)
    f. Flaccid paralysis with loss of reflexes
    g. Possible involvement of facial, extraocular, labial, lingual, pharyngeal, and laryngeal muscles
    h. Involvement of intercostal and phrenic nerves (breathlessness in vocalization; shallow, irregular respirations)
22. Symptomatically, often with assisted ventilation
23. Clostridium tetani
24. immune status

25. Tetanus immune globulin and tetanus toxoid
26. The ingestion of spores or vegetative cells of *Clostridium botulinum* and the subsequent release of the toxin from organisms colonizing the gastrointestinal tract; inadequately cooked or improperly canned food, honey, light or dark corn syrup
27. a. Constipation
    b. Generalized weakness and a decrease in spontaneous movements
    c. Deep tendon reflexes usually diminished or absent
    d. Cranial nerve deficits commonly present (loss of head control, difficulty feeding, weak cry, and reduced gag reflex)
28. Clinical history, physical examination, and laboratory detection of toxin or the organism in the patient's blood or stool
29. With the immediate intravenous administration of botulism immune globulin
30. motor vehicle crashes
31. a. Complete or partial paralysis of the lower extremities
    b. No functional use of any of the four extremities
32. a. Maintenance of airway patency
    b. Prevention of complications
    c. Maintenance of function
33. deep vein thrombosis, pulmonary embolus

Applying Critical Thinking to the Nursing Practice

A.

1. Risk for Injury related to physical disability, neuromuscular impairment, and perceptual and cognitive impairment
2. Angela will experience no physical injury.
3. a. Educate the family to provide a safe physical environment.
   b. Educate the family to select toys appropriate for age and ability.
   c. Encourage sufficient rest to reduce fatigue and decrease risk of injuries.

d. Use safety restraints when the child is in a chair or vehicle.
   e. Provide the child who is prone to falls with protective helmet and enforce its use to prevent head injuries.
   f. Institute seizure precautions for the susceptible child.
4. The family will provide a safe environment for Angela by… (add something specific, eg, family will have sturdy furniture that does not slip to prevent falls).

B.

1. a. Infant will not experience damage to the myelomeningocele sac.
   b. Infant will not experience complications.
   c. Family will receive support and education.
2. a. The myelomeningocele sac sustains no damage.
   b. The child exhibits no evidence of complications.
   c. The family members discuss their feelings and concerns and participate in the infant's care.

C.

1. Helping the child and family cope with a chronic, progressive, incapacitating disease; helping design a program that will afford maximal independence and reduce the predictable and preventable disabilities associated with the disorder; and helping the child and family deal constructively with the limitations the disease imposes on their daily lives
2. Genetic counseling

D.

1. a. Clinical manifestations
   b. Cerebrospinal fluid analysis
   c. Electromyography findings
2. Gabapentin

E.

1. Indirect trauma caused by sudden hyperflexion or hyperextension of the neck, often combined with a rotational force
2. Preparing the child and family to live at home and function as independently as possible.